HOLD
The Fat, Sugar & Salt

GOLDIE SILVERMAN
and
JACQUELINE WILLIAMS

Illustrated by Mary Mietzelfeld

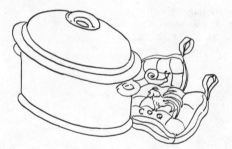

A PERIGEE BOOK

Perigee Books
are published by
The Putnam Publishing Group
200 Madison Avenue
New York, New York 10016

LIBRARY OF CONGRESS CATALOGING IN PUBLICATION DATA

Silverman, Goldie.
   Hold the fat, sugar & salt.

1. Sugar-free diet—Recipes.   2. Low-fat diet—Recipes.
3. Salt-free diet—Recipes.   I. Williams, Jacqueline.
II. Title.
RM237.85.W55   1984   641.5′632   84-7052
ISBN 0-399-51073-7

Cover design copyright 1984 by Terrence Fehr

First Perigee printing, 1984
Printed in the United States of America
20 19 18 17 16 15 14 13 12

Contents

PART I

Preface

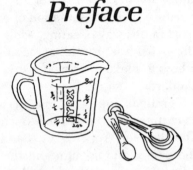

Good health is in. It's hardly news that you should decrease the amounts of the three villains—salt, sugar and fat—in your diet.

Making the decision to change your eating habits is easy. Adopting new habits is harder. Many people who have tried to cut out salt, sugar and fat gave up when they found their meals tasteless and boring. They had the right idea but they didn't know how to bring their good intentions to the table.

In the beginning it was difficult for us, too, but we had no choice; a heart problem in the family required us to change our diet. So we had to stay with the new pattern of cooking, and little by little we learned to substitute ingredients, to adapt to new ways and to use unfamiliar foods. Suddenly we found ourselves regarded as experts in the field, being asked to share recipes, write a cookbook and even teach classes.

Our students taught us a lot! We realized that people couldn't adjust to a whole new style of eating overnight. They wanted to continue eating familiar foods, and they needed time to allow their taste buds to accept even gradual changes.

We learned that different people had differing goals and needs; some wanted to cut out all salt or all fats, while others wanted only to reduce their consumption of each. Some were just getting started in this way of eating, while others were old hands looking for new ideas. But all agreed that they wanted instructions on how to make their own everyday recipes conform to new standards.

We devised a gradual approach that began with cutting down and led to cutting out. We learned to select the healthier ingredients. (The charts in Appendixes A and B, which compare the fat, cholesterol and sodium and the caloric content and nutrients of some common foods, will show you why we made our choices.) We took familiar recipes and substituted ingredients to reduce salt, sugar and fat without drastically changing the recipes. We developed a group of basics (stocks, sauces, seasonings and salad dressings) that can be the foundation for many dishes. In some cases we created new ingredients to take the place of less healthful ones. All the while we were tasting, tasting, tasting to guarantee that our meals would remain enjoyable.

Our students convinced us that we should share our methods as well as our recipes. There are lots of cookbooks around, they said, but none of them deals with adapting familiar recipes and making them healthier. So this book was born. In the first section of *Hold the Fat, Sugar & Salt* we show you how to adjust and how to substitute in your own recipes; this will enable you to decrease the fat, sugar and salt in your diet gradually, without giving up all your favorite foods. In the second half we share our own adapted recipes, from family fare to gourmet cuisine. At the same time we introduce a few new foods that our families find especially delectable.

How We Cook

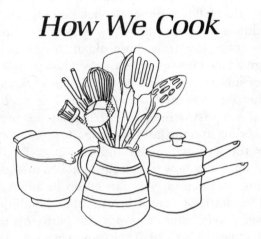

Most of us are fluent in the language of cooking: that is, we can follow the steps of a recipe as it is given without having to stop and think about the directions. If the recipe says "stir," "blend" or "mix," we automatically reach for our favorite spoon or spatula and move it around the bowl until all the separate ingredients are combined into one homogeneous whole. If a recipe tells us to cook a food to a certain stage, we know that we must watch our onions until they are golden or our ground beef until "no trace of pink remains." But if a recipe says "season to taste," you probably reach for the salt shaker first, while we are aware of many other options.

Learning to cook our way does not mean learning a whole new kitchen language. Most of the steps you will take in preparing a recipe will still be the same. You will chop, stir and simmer as before. But for a few directions, you will act differently. So if the recipe says "season to taste," you will have lots of other methods for developing added flavor without adding salt.

Which standard instructions need to be changed in your

own familiar recipes? We have listed them in the left column of the chart that follows, under the heading Old Instructions. In the column on the right, we present new directions to follow whenever you read those old instructions. In many cases we give you a choice of new directions, so that you have a variety of substitutes; if you don't like one method, you may find another that suits you better. Where it is applicable, we have listed our instructions in order, with the first one the least demanding and the last requiring the greatest change. At the end of this section we give you our recipe for Beef Stew, which demonstrates how to use our methods in your kitchen.

Using our techniques, you can go on to adapt your own recipes. The charts of "Fat, Cholesterol and Sodium Content of Common Foods" and "Calories and Nutrients of Selected Foods" on pages 152–155 will help you select substitute ingredients knowledgeably. Make your changes little by little and give yourself time to get used to them. At the same time you can try some of our favorites that we have included in the second section of this book.

OLD INSTRUCTIONS	NEW INSTRUCTIONS
fry, sauté, brown	**1.** Reduce the amount of fat. If the recipe calls for ¼ cup, try 2 tablespoons.

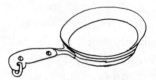

—or—

2. Halve the amount of fat; replace the missing fat with an equal amount of our unsalted, defatted stocks, which we tell you how to prepare on pages 25 through 28. Work toward a minimun amount of fat (½ teaspoon) with stock.

—or—

3. Cook in one of our unsalted, defatted stocks. Heat 1 to 2 tablespoons stock to medium high; add vegetables or meat. Stir quickly until tender-crisp, allowing most of the liquid to evaporate. When cooking vegetables, do not

let too much liquid collect in the pan.
Raise the heat so liquid evaporates, or the
vegetables will be soft instead of crisp.

—or—

4. Use a heavy iron skillet. Put 1 teaspoon oil in it, wipe skillet clean with
paper towels and then heat. Brown
using only the oil left in the skillet.

—or—

5. Use a nonstick frying pan and no
fat.

—or—

6. Brown on a rack under the broiler.
Fat can be discarded.

OLD INSTRUCTIONS	NEW INSTRUCTIONS

pour melted fat over

1. Brush fat on with a pastry brush.
(You'll be surprised to see how little
you need.)

2. Mix equal parts fat and unsalted,
defatted stock (pp. 25–28). Then pour.

OLD INSTRUCTIONS	NEW INSTRUCTIONS

season to taste

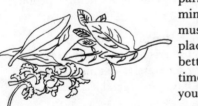

1. Whenever possible, use fresh herbs:
parsley, thyme, basil, sage, tarragon,
mint and chives. Fresh parsley is a
must for us. It is available in most
places year-round. Frozen herbs are
better than dried. Substitute three
times as much chopped fresh herb as
your recipe calls for dried; use frozen
as you would fresh.

GREMOLATA: Mix 3 tablespoons finely chopped fresh parsley, 1 tablespoon grated lemon peel and 1 teaspoon finely
chopped garlic. Sprinkle on cooked meat or vegetable dishes.

2. When you must use dried herbs and spices, freshen them by crushing them in a mortar and pestle or with the back of a spoon.

3. Try new seasonings. Take a chance on something on the grocer's shelf that you've never used before. Begin with ¼ teaspoon of a spice or an herb, aromatic bitters or one of our shake-on mixes. Taste and add.

4. Correct tartness: A little grated carrot or parsnip will make tomato-based sauces and soups sweeter, less tart.

5. Use freshly grated nutmeg. Keep the grater on the table instead of a salt shaker. Sprinkle on asparagus.

6. Add a "kick" to meat, vegetables, salads and grains with dry mustard, ¼ teaspoon at a time.

7. Experiment with flavored mustards. Look for salt-free varieties, but if you can't find them, one teaspoon of Dijon mustard (containing 70 milligrams of sodium) is not much salt in a recipe for four.

8. Try new flavor combinations. Cumin, tumeric and coriander, together or separately, add an exotic Eastern flavor to vegetables, grains or chicken.

ALGERIAN RICE: Mix two cups hot cooked rice with ½ teaspoon coriander, ¼ teaspoon cumin and ¼ cup raisins that have been soaked in ¼ cup sherry.

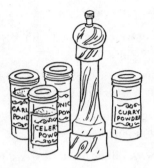

9. Use flavored vinegar in soups, sauces and salad dressings or over vegetables. Flavored vinegars require less oil for vinaigrette.

10. Add 1 tablespoon sherry to clear broth.

OLD INSTRUCTIONS	NEW INSTRUCTIONS
add onion salt, garlic salt, celery salt, or all-purpose seasoning	**1.** Use onion or garlic powder, or celery seeds. **2.** Use one of our seasoning mixes.

NOTE: It's the sodium in salt that's the villain! A tablespoon of salt contains 6000 milligrams of sodium; a tablespoon of soy sauce contains 2000; a tablespoon of Worcestershire sauce contains about 240 milligrams; and a tablespoon of aromatic bitters contains only .48 milligrams of sodium.

OLD INSTRUCTIONS	NEW INSTRUCTIONS
add MSG (monosodium glutamate)	Leave it out! It's nothing but sodium!
use canned broth or bouillon cube	Use one of our basic stocks. (pp. 25-28)

Freeze stock in ice cube trays; remove and store in a plastic bag in the freezer. Use these frozen "stock cubes" for seasoning or sautéing.

OLD INSTRUCTIONS	NEW INSTRUCTIONS

cook in salted water

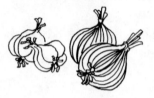

1. Cook rice in water seasoned with one tablespoon vinegar.

2. Put a garlic clove or a piece of onion in water for cooking pasta.

3. Add a sprig of mint or a small onion to boiling potatoes.

4. Add caraway, dill or mustard seeds to water for cooking vegetables.

OLD INSTRUCTIONS	NEW INSTRUCTIONS

add canned tomato sauce (high in salt)

1. Buy no-salt-added tomato sauce.

2. Use tomato paste or tomato puree (no-salt-added) and dilute with water or stock to bring it up to the right quantity.

3. Use our recipe for homemade tomato sauce (see p. 32).

QUICK SUPPER: Stir leftover cooked vegetables, beans or meat into one of our tomato sauces. Heat and serve over hot cooked pasta, rice or baked potato.

OLD INSTRUCTIONS	NEW INSTRUCTIONS

use whole milk

1. Use 2% or 1% milk (see Chart page 152).

2. Use skim or nonfat milk.

3. Use dry nonfat milk, reconstituted.

OLD INSTRUCTIONS	NEW INSTRUCTIONS
use heavy cream	Use one of our substitute cream recipes (see p. 40).
use sour cream	**1.** Use a tofu topping; check our recipes.
	2. Use one of our substitute sour creams (see p. 41).
add mayonnaise	Use our tofu mayonnaise (see p. 36).

OLD INSTRUCTIONS	NEW INSTRUCTIONS
use hard cheese (cheddar, Swiss or Parmesan)	**1.** Choose low-fat cheese, such as mozzarella or sapsago.
	2. Combine cheeses; for example, mix half Parmesan and half sapsago to use on spaghetti.
	3. Use low-sodium cheese and cut down on fat in other ingredients.

Yellow or hard cheeses (as opposed to cottage or curd cheeses) are high in fat, cholesterol and sodium; ordinary cheddar cheese contains 9.4 grams of fat per ounce, 30 milligrams of cholesterol and 176 milligrams of sodium (see Chart p. 152). That's more in each category than you would get in an ounce of chicken, fish or even lean beef. For our recipes we have chosen cheeses the fat content of which is under 5 grams per ounce, and we have used them sparingly. Unfortunately, most low-fat cheeses are high in sodium, and vice versa. When you adapt your own recipes, you will have to adjust these according to your own needs. Read the label on cheeses carefully; if one has more than 5 grams of fat per ounce, it isn't low fat. If you choose low-fat cheese, be certain the other ingredients in your recipe are low in sodium; if you choose low-sodium cheese, be sure the rest of your ingredients are low in fat. If you can find a good cheese that is both low-fat and low-sodium, by all means use it.

OLD INSTRUCTIONS	NEW INSTRUCTIONS
use ground beef	**1.** Use low-fat ground beef.
	2. Use ground veal.
	3. Use ground turkey.
	4. Cut down on amount of meat; use meat as a seasoning and increase vegetables.

OLD INSTRUCTIONS	NEW INSTRUCTIONS
use whole eggs	**1.** Use two egg whites for one egg.
	2. Use one whole egg and two egg whites for two eggs.

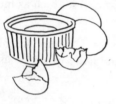

OLD INSTRUCTIONS	NEW INSTRUCTIONS
add cream soup or canned white sauce	Use one of our white sauces (see pp. 29–31).

OLD INSTRUCTIONS	NEW INSTRUCTIONS
thicken with flour and butter	**1.** Reduce liquid by rapid boiling.
	2. Thicken with cornstarch, rice or potato flours, or nonfat dry milk.

OLD INSTRUCTIONS	NEW INSTRUCTIONS
use sugar or honey	**1.** Halve the amount of sugar in cookies or cakes.
	2. Increase the amount of extract (vanilla, almond or orange) in cakes or cookies by ¼ teaspoon to compensate for halved or reduced sugar.

3. Use fruit juice concentrate (1 table-spoon equals 1 teaspoon sugar).

Juice concentrate in a pie filling will take the place of all the sugar.

4. Use unsweetened white grape juice (2 tablespoons equal 1 teaspoon sugar) when poaching fruit.

5. Substitute fruit juice for honey in Middle Eastern lamb and chicken dishes.

6. Use pureed fruit or dried fruit as a sweetener.

Stir applesauce, fruit juice or banana puree into rice pudding. Substitute dried fruit for candied fruit in fruit cake and holiday recipes.

7. Substitute sweet wine for water when preparing fruit or flavoring a stew.

OLD INSTRUCTIONS

sweeten to taste

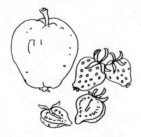

NEW INSTRUCTIONS

1. Add dried fruit to cereals.

2. Make your own breakfast yogurt by stirring fresh fruit, cereal, juice concentrate and plain nonfat yogurt together.

3. Sprinkle fruit-flavored liqueurs over fresh fruit.

4. Enhance the flavor of baked goods by adding grated orange or lemon rind.

5. Use grated sweet vegetables such as carrots, sweet potatoes and parsnips in casseroles that are too tart.

Mexican, Italian and Greek dishes based on tomatoes often call for sugar; try using grated vegetables instead.

---

6. Use cinnamon, ginger, nutmeg, cardamom.

7. Add instant nonfat dry milk to breads, puddings and creamy sweet sauces.

NOTE: Juices work best in sauces or cooked dishes. If you try them with baked goods, you *must* omit an equal volume of liquid from your recipe to compensate for added volume of sweeteners.

OLD INSTRUCTIONS	NEW INSTRUCTIONS
use one package fruit gelatin	Use unflavored gelatin and fruit juices.

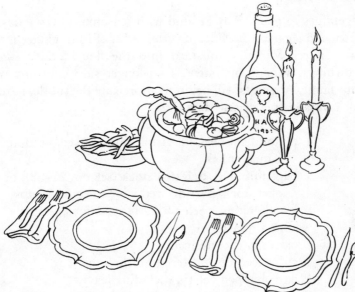

Beef Stew Our Way

Chunks of beef cooked in a rich sauce, whether you call it stew or Bourguignonne, is a dish that everyone knows how to make. Just to show you how our methods work, we have adapted this classic recipe to our new standards.

In the past you probably began by tossing the beef chunks in flour seasoned with salt and other spices. Then you browned the chunks in ¼ cup hot fat (450 to 500 calories), added vegetables and water, and simmered the whole rich mix for one to two hours.

Now you can make the same delicious stew with no salt and reduced fat. Start by drying the meat chunks with paper towels and skipping the flour. We brown ours under the broiler, but you can use any of the methods we describe under New Instructions. Instead of adding plain water to the stew, choose a flavorful stock or wine. Use the same meat and vegetables that you have always used, but increase the proportion of vegetables to meat. Play around with seasonings. Try a dash of wine vinegar in the stock or grate a bit of fresh ginger into your sauce. Mix dry mustard into the flour (added *after* browning). When your stew is no longer salty and greasy, your family or guests will begin to appreciate the subtle, natural flavors of this classic dish.

1	pound lean beef, all visible fat removed, cut into 1-inch cubes
2	cups unsalted, defatted stock (see pp. 25–28), or part stock/part dry red wine to equal 2 cups
8	small onions, peeled, or 2 large onions, peeled and quartered
1–2	cloves garlic, minced
1	cup sliced or quartered mushrooms
1	cup chopped celery, including leaves
1	cup sliced carrots, scrubbed but not peeled
½	teaspoon dry mustard
2	tablespoons flour
1	tablespoon chopped fresh parsley
1	or 2 bay leaves
6	peppercorns
6	whole cloves
½	teaspoon Worcestershire sauce, or bitters to taste
4	medium potatoes, scrubbed and quartered
1	large parsnip, scrubbed and sliced

Brown the meat using one of our methods. Drain beef on paper towels. If your stew will cook in the same pan, wipe the pan to remove fat. Heat 1 to 2 tablespoons stock in a Dutch oven or deep stew pan. Add onions and cook for 3 to 4 minutes. Add garlic, mushrooms, celery and carrots; cook for 3 to 4 minutes more. Mix dry mustard into flour. Remove pan from heat.

Sprinkle flour over vegetables and stir until thoroughly mixed. Return pan to the burner. Blend in remaining stock or substitute liquid, remaining seasonings and Worcestershire sauce or bitters. Return meat to the pan; add potatoes and parsnips. Bring mixture to a boil; then simmer, covered, for 1½ to 2 hours or cook, covered, in a 325-degree oven for same amount of time. Check occasionally to be sure stew is not drying out; add stock or wine as necessary.

Makes 4 servings.

Basics

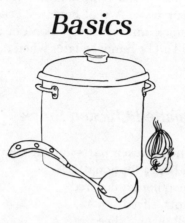

These are the indispensable low-salt, low-fat, low-sugar stocks, sauces and seasonings that we substitute for the other kind of ingredient in traditional recipes. Use these basics as suggested in New Instructions to make your own favorites conform to new standards or use them in the recipes in the second section of *Hold the Fat, Sugar & Salt*.

STOCKS

A delicious stock is not only the base for many soups and sauces, it is also the major substitute for oil in cooking. We cannot overemphasize the importance of good stocks, which depend on good ingredients. For that reason the cook should constantly be aware of potential ingredients for stock. The water in which vegetables were cooked, the juices drained or rendered from chicken dishes, marinades from meats and the cooked bones from poultry or roasts should all be stored in the freezer for the stockpot. When you are ready to make stock, be sure to add these goodies. Chicken parts can be unusable ones like wing tips, necks, skin and bones. Vegetables may vary according to your taste. A veal bone, especially the knuckle, will enrich the stock immeasurably. Don't be concerned about adding fat; it will all be removed later when the stock is chilled and strained.

Unsalted, Defatted Chicken Stock

     2–3 pounds chicken parts and/or trimmings
     1–2 veal bones (optional)
        1 large onion, quartered
        2 carrots, sliced
        1 small turnip, sliced
     1–2 celery ribs, with leaves
     4–6 whole peppercorns
        1 cup mushroom stems, chopped
     2–3 fresh parsley stems
     1–2 cloves garlic, minced
     1–2 sprigs fresh thyme, or ½ teaspoon dried
             ¼–½-inch piece fresh ginger (optional)
    8–10 cups water
             bones and appropriate vegetable and meat juices
                saved for stock (see p. 25)

Place all ingredients in a large soup kettle. Bring to a boil; cover and simmer for 3 to 4 hours. Remove and discard chicken and vegetables. Cool and then chill stock. Remove congealed fat and discard; strain the stock through a double thickness of cheesecloth. Stock may be frozen.

   Makes about 2 quarts.

NOTE: To remove fat in a hurry, pour stock or pan drippings from meat into a glass jar or plastic container. Set container in refrigerator for 20 to 30 minutes and let the fat rise to the top. Remove it carefully with a spoon or a baster. A fat separator is a good invest-ment; it allows you to pour the good, defatted meat juice or stock out from under a layer of fat without waiting for it to solidify.

Vegetable Stock

The simplest vegetable stock is made by saving all the juices from cooking vegetables and all the trimmings from preparing them (bits of carrots and celery, tough broccoli stems, peelings from potatoes, parsnips and carrots). Keep a plastic container in your freezer for accumulating vegetable leftovers, juices and washed trimmings. When you have collected several cups' worth, put them in a large soup kettle; add more seasonings, onion, garlic, thyme, parsley or dill, and simmer for 1½ hours. Strain the stock, cool and refrigerate.

Those who like more specific direction can do this:

```
  2    onions, chopped
2–3    cloves garlic, minced
  1    cup mushrooms
2–3    celery ribs with leaves, cut up
  1    bay leaf
1–2    cups potato peelings
  2    carrots, chopped
  1    turnip, chopped
  1    small tomato, cut up
 ¼     cup fresh parsley, chopped
3–4    whole peppercorns
6–8    cups water
```

Combine vegetables, seasonings and water in a large soup kettle. Cover and simmer for 1–1½ hours. Strain, cool and refrigerate. Stock may be frozen.

Makes about 2 quarts.

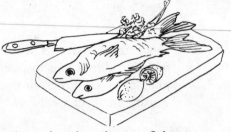

Fish Stock

Fish stock is useful as a base for chowders or fish sauces. Canned or bottled clam juice is often suggested as a substitute for fish stock, but it is extremely high in sodium.

Most fishmongers will gladly part with their extra fish trimmings. Just make certain they are fresh and avoid oily fish like salmon or black cod.

2	pounds fish trimmings (heads and bones)
1	teaspoon margarine, no salt added
1	large onion, chopped
4–6	mushrooms, thinly sliced
1	clove garlic, unpeeled
1	carrot, sliced thin
1	rib celery with leaves, chopped
2–3	green onions, finely chopped
6–8	peppercorns
6–8	parsley stems
2–3	sprigs fresh thyme, or ½ teaspoon dried
1	bay leaf
½	cup dry white wine
5–6	cups water, or to cover

Wash fish several times in cold water. Melt margarine in a large kettle; add vegetables and fish and cook over low heat until vegetables are soft—about 5 minutes. Add remaining ingredients and water to cover; bring to a boil. Partially cover the kettle and simmer for 30 minutes. Strain, pressing all juices from vegetables and fish. This stock keeps for about a week in the refrigerator, or it may be frozen.

Makes about 4 cups.

SAUCES

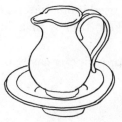

Basic White Sauce with Milk (Béchamel)

Vegetables steeped in hot milk add flavor to this versatile sauce, which can replace the butter-flour-milk white sauce in any of your recipes. It also forms the base of a salt-free cheese sauce that in its turn can dress vegetables, open-face sandwiches, fish, macaroni or baked potatoes.

> 1 cup nonfat milk
> small piece of onion (about 1 tablespoon)
> 2 tablespoons grated carrot
> ⅛ teaspoon freshly grated nutmeg
> ⅛ teaspoon white pepper
> 2 tablespoons instant nonfat dry milk
> 1 tablespoon cornstarch or arrowroot
> 2 tablespoons flour

In a small saucepan combine milk, onion, carrot, nutmeg and pepper. Bring to a boil, then cover, remove from heat and allow to steep for ten minutes. Pour the warm milk through a strainer, pressing down on the vegetables to obtain all the juices. Let cool. Combine dry milk, cornstarch or arrowroot and flour. Add one or two tablespoons cooled milk to the dry mixture and stir to a smooth paste. Return the milk to the saucepan, add the flour paste and stir over medium heat until mixture boils and thickens.

If sauce will not be used immediately, cover and refrigerate. Cold sauce will thicken; thin with a little flavored cooking juice, wine or stock.

Makes about 1 cup; recipe is easily doubled.

Cheese Sauce

     1 cup Béchamel Sauce
    ½ cup grated low-sodium cheese
     1 teaspoon Dijon-style mustard, no salt added
    ¼ teaspoon paprika
  2–3 drops liquid hot pepper seasoning

Heat Béchamel Sauce; add cheese, mustard, paprika and seasoning. Stir over medium heat until cheese melts and blends.

Makes about 1½ cups.

Basic White Sauce with Stock (Velouté)

Velouté Sauce, made with a rich stock, is a flavorful topping for fish, potatoes or vegetables. Though it takes more time to prepare than Béchamel, it can be made in large quantities and frozen.

     1 tablespoon salt-free margarine
     1 cup plus 1 tablespoon unsalted defatted stock
         (see p. 26)
     1 tablespoon instant nonfat dry milk
     2 tablespoons flour

Melt margarine in a small nonstick saucepan. Add 1 tablespoon stock. Combine dry milk and flour; stir into margarine to make a roux. Cook for 1 minute or until roux thickens. Slowly pour in remaining stock and mix until roux and liquid are well blended. Cook over medium heat, stirring constantly, until mixture boils and begins to thicken. Reduce to a slow simmer for 15 minutes, stirring occasionally. If stock will not be used immediately, cover and refrigerate.

Makes 1 cup.

Demiglacé Sauce

Demiglacé Sauce is syrupy when hot and jellied when cold. In traditional French cooking it is used to impart a special flavor to rich sauces. When you have time, make a batch (it freezes well). Use it on Chicken Bourguignonne (see p. 76).

> 2 cups rich gelatinous unsalted, defatted stock
> (see pp. 25–28)
> 2 shallots or ¼ small onion, finely chopped
> 1 tablespoon flour
> 3–4 mushroom stems
> 1–2 parsley stems
> 1 bay leaf
> bits of tomato peelings (optional)
> 2–3 peppercorns

Heat 2 tablespoons stock and slowly cook shallots or onion until golden brown. Add flour and stir until well mixed and flour begins to brown. (Add extra stock 1 teaspoon at a time if mixture seems dry.) When flour is brown, add remaining stock and other ingredients. Bring to a boil and simmer, uncovered, for 20 minutes. Strain before using.

If you have a thinner stock, follow the same method, but simmer longer over very low heat, about 30 minutes.

Makes about 1½ cups.

TOMATO SAUCE

Both our recipes for tomato sauce use canned tomato puree, which should have no salt added. Of course you can make your own puree by simmering cut-up fresh tomatoes until thick and then straining out the peel and seeds. If you're a gardener with a plentiful harvest of tomatoes, you can puree your surplus and freeze it in measured portions.

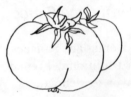

Piquant Tomato Sauce

        ¾ cup finely chopped onion
      2–4 cloves garlic, minced
        1 cup unsalted, defatted stock (see pp. 25–28)
        3 cups tomato puree, no salt added or homemade
        ½ cup finely chopped fresh parsley
        ¼ cup fresh or frozen minced basil leaves,
              or 2 teaspoons dried
        1 tablespoon grated orange rind
        2 teaspoons fresh lemon or lime juice
           freshly ground pepper

Cook onion and garlic in 2 tablespoons stock just until vegetables are tender. Add remaining ingredients and simmer for 20 to 30 minutes. Taste and adjust seasoning.

Makes about 4 cups.

Tomato Wine Sauce

  1   shallot, finely chopped
1–2   cloves garlic, minced
  1   teaspoon olive oil
  1   small carrot, grated
  2   cups tomato puree, no salt added
¼–½   cup red or white wine
  1   teaspoon paprika
2–3   fresh basil leaves, minced, or 1 teaspoon dried
  ¼   teaspoon dry mustard
       dash red pepper flakes (optional)

Cook shallot and garlic in oil; add carrot and cook until soft. Stir in puree, wine and seasonings. Simmer for 25 to 35 minutes. Taste and adjust seasoning.

Makes about 2½ cups.

For a thicker sauce, puree half or all of either our Piquant Tomato Sauce or our Tomato Wine Sauce in blender or food processor.

SALAD DRESSINGS

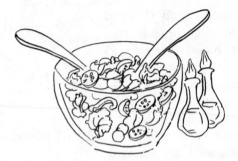

Most of us have a favorite oil or creamy salad dressing. When the waitperson rattles off the list—French, Italian or oil and vinegar—we know exactly what we want.

When you choose a salad dressing, you can have what you want and still practice adapting and substituting to reduce the salt, fat and sugar in your diet. Begin gradually by tossing your salad with a small amount of dressing rather than pouring a large amount over the top. Then you can cut down on the oil in the dressing and replace the volume with an equal amount of a new ingredient, such as tofu or a very rich un-salted defatted stock. Use the herbs and seasonings you like, but also try new combinations and substitutes, such as our seasoning mixes. Finally, use the freshest possible ingredients in your salads and arrange them attractively to make them delicious and eye appealing.

Basic Vinaigrette

    2 teaspoons olive oil
   ¼ cup Unsalted, Defatted Chicken Stock (see p. 26)
   1 tablespoon sherry vinegar
1–2 cloves garlic, mashed

¼ teaspoon dry mustard
1 tablespoon finely chopped parsley
1–2 leaves fresh basil, minced, or ½ teaspoon dried
freshly ground pepper to taste

Combine all ingredients in a glass jar. Shake well. Allow to stand 2 hours before using.
Makes 4 servings.

Fruited Vinegar Salad Dressing

Flavored vinegars combined with fruit juice make a pleasant low-calorie dressing for a salad that combines greens with sweet vegetables, such as fresh or frozen peas and/or grated carrot.

4 tablespoons white wine or rice vinegar
2 cloves garlic, peeled
sprig of fresh parsley
¼–½ teaspoon Dijon-style mustard
juice of 1 medium orange
freshly ground pepper to taste
half an orange, peeled and cut into small pieces

Combine all ingredients except orange pieces in a glass jar. Shake well. Add orange pieces just before serving.
Makes four servings.

Vegetable-Herb Salad Dressing

1 cup canned vegetable juice cocktail, no salt added
or reduced salt
¼ cup red wine vinegar

1 teaspoon frozen apple juice concentrate
⅛ teaspoon ground cumin
¼ teaspoon crumbled dried oregano
¼ teaspoon ground celery seed
1 clove garlic, mashed
　 freshly ground pepper to taste
　 dash Worcestershire sauce
2 teaspoons cornstarch
2 tablespoons cold water
2 tablespoons minced chives

In a small pan bring to a simmer the vegetable juice, vinegar, apple juice concentrate, cumin, oregano, celery seed, garlic, pepper and Worcestershire sauce. Dissolve the cornstarch in the cold water, then add to dressing. Slowly bring mixture to a boil. Cook one minute, reduce heat and stir until thickened.

Remove from heat, add chives and adjust seasonings. This dressing will keep for 2 weeks if stored in a covered container in the refrigerator.

Makes about 1½ cups.

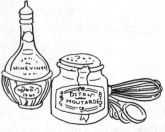

Tofu Mayonnaise

Tofu is a food that has come a long way, from China in the year 2000 B.C., through Japan and on to North America, where in 1982 an Orthodox Jewish rabbi granted his *hecksher* (certificate of Kosher standards) to a tofu processing plant near Seattle. Tofu mayonnaise can be substituted in many familiar salad dressings or sandwich spreads; our variations should be just a starting point for your own experiments.

 1 cup tofu, well drained
 1 tablespoon rice vinegar
 1 teaspoon Dijon-style mustard, no salt added
 ¼ teaspoon dry mustard
   white pepper to taste

Puree tofu in a food processor or blender. Add remaining ingredients. Cover and let stand for 1 hour before using.
 Makes about 1 cup.

VARIATIONS: Each variation is prepared in the same way: In a small bowl combine tofu mayonnaise and remaining ingredients. Cover and let stand for several hours for flavors to blend.

THOUSAND-ISLAND DRESSING

  1 cup tofu mayonnaise
  3 tablespoons tomato paste, no salt added
 1½ tablespoons white wine vinegar, or rice vinegar
  2 tablespoons finely chopped celery
  2 tablespoons finely chopped green pepper
  ¼ teaspoon sweet paprika
  2 hard-boiled eggs, whites only, diced

SEAFOOD SALAD DRESSING

  1 cup tofu mayonnaise
  3 tablespoons tomato paste, no salt added
 1½ tablespoons white wine vinegar, or rice vinegar
  2 tablespoons finely chopped green pepper
  2 tablespoons finely chopped green onion
  1 teaspoon lemon juice

POTATO SALAD MAYONNAISE

     ½ cup tofu mayonnaise
   2–3 sprigs fresh dill, or ¼ teaspoon dry dill weed
     2 green onions, finely chopped
     1 teaspoon finely chopped fresh parsley

This dressing can also be served over boiled potatoes or as a topping for baked potatoes.

GREEN GODDESS SALAD DRESSING

     1 cup tofu mayonnaise
     ¼ cup low-fat cottage cheese
     1 tablespoon tarragon vinegar
     1 tablespoon garlic wine vinegar
     2 tablespoons chopped parsley
     2 teaspoons crumbled dried tarragon leaves
     2 tablespoons fresh chopped chives, or 2 teaspoons
       dried
   1–2 green onions, finely chopped, or 2 teaspoons
       onion powder

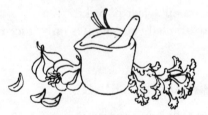

PESTOLIKE SALAD DRESSING

     2 cups fresh basil leaves, coarsely chopped and
       tightly packed
     ½ cup tofu mayonnaise

1   clove garlic, minced
1   teaspoon finely chopped walnuts
1   tablespoon olive oil
    freshly ground pepper to taste

Serve over hot pasta or hot or cold vegetables.

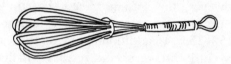

Sweet Tofu Topping

We call it a topping, but we often serve this sweetened whipped tofu as a dessert all by itself.

¾   cup tofu
1   tablespoon frozen juice concentrate
⅛   teaspoon almond flavoring
½   cup sliced ripe banana

Beat or whip the tofu to a smooth puree. Add juice concentrate, flavoring and banana slices and continue to beat until the mix is thick and smooth. Serve as a sauce over fruit. Flavors will intensify if sauce is made ahead and chilled.
    Makes about 1 cup.

SUBSTITUTE CREAMS

Do you automatically reject recipes that call for whipped or sour cream because you have no low-fat substitute? Our "creams" will make those recipes acceptable.

Each group of cream substitutes is arranged in order of diminishing fat; in other words, the first one in each group contains the most fat. None of the substitutes contains added sodium; however, the cottage cheese–based "creams" are high in sodium because cottage cheese is high in sodium (see Chart pp. 152–153). In addition to having the least amount of fat, the dry-curd cottage cheese recipes will have the least amount of sodium because this cheese is unsalted.

Substitute Whipping Cream

These "creams" can be used in any vegetable dishes and in fish, chicken or pasta recipes that use heavy cream. They hold up when cooked, and in gelatins. Flavored with fruit concentrates or pureed fruit, they make delicious toppings for plain cakes and fruit.

> skim-milk ricotta "cream"
> low-fat (2%) cottage cheese "cream"
> dry-curd cottage cheese "cream"

The basic recipe is the same for all three: Mix 2 cups cheese (ricotta, cottage cheese or dry curd) with ½ cup plain low-fat or nonfat yogurt. Using a food processor, a blender or an electric mixer, beat or puree until very smooth. The mixture should not be grainy, although the dry cottage cheese "cream" will retain a touch of graininess. Pour the "cream" into a bowl, cover and let stand at room temperature for four to six hours to allow fermentation to take place. The "cream" will be as thick as whipped cream and light in texture. Refrigerate the "cream" in a covered bowl for several hours before using. "Cream" keeps for seven to ten days.

Makes about 2½ cups.

Substitute Sour Cream

- 1 cup low-fat (2%) cottage cheese pureed with ¼ cup plain low-fat or nonfat yogurt
- 1 cup plain low-fat or nonfat yogurt
- 1 cup dry-curd cottage cheese pureed with 2 tablespoons skim-milk buttermilk and ½ teaspoon lemon juice

OUR SEASONING MIXES

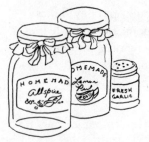

When we first began cooking without salt, we liked to have a shake-on mix at the table to satisfy the old habit of reaching for a shaker and to enable us to perk up bland foods. Now we keep a mix around just to provide for guests who automatically shake before tasting.

Packed in attractive jars or shakers, the mixes are lovely gifts.

General directions: Mix all ingredients in blender or food processor. Store in glass shaker.

All-Purpose Seasoning # 1

    1 tablespoon garlic powder
    1 teaspoon dried basil
    1 teaspoon dried marjoram
    1 teaspoon dried thyme
    1 teaspoon dried parsley
    1 teaspoon dried savory
    1 teaspoon onion powder
    1 teaspoon ground white pepper
    1 teaspoon ground mace (optional)

All-Purpose Seasoning # 2

    1 tablespoon parsley flakes
    1 tablespoon tarragon leaves
    1½ teaspoons oregano leaves
    1½ teaspoons dill weed
    1 teaspoon celery seed

Hot and Spicy Seasoning

    2 tablespoons turmeric
    1½ tablespoons coriander
    1 teaspoon cayenne
    2 teaspoons dry mustard
    2 teaspoons cumin
    2 teaspoons cinnamon
    2 teaspoons ground ginger
    1 teaspoon ground white pepper

Italian Seasoning

    1 tablespoon dried basil
    1 tablespoon dried oregano
    1 tablespoon dried parsley
    1 teaspoon dried thyme
    1 teaspoon dried marjoram
   ½ teaspoon paprika
   ¼ teaspoon red pepper flakes

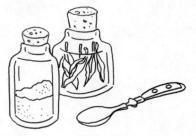

Poultry Seasoning

    2 teaspoons marjoram
    2 teaspoons dried sage
    1 teaspoon dried rosemary
    1 teaspoon dried thyme
    1 teaspoon oregano
   ½ teaspoon ground nutmeg
   ½ teaspoon ground white pepper

Vegetable Seasoning

    4 tablespoons dried parsley
    1 tablespoon dried basil
    1 teaspoon dried mint
    1 teaspoon dried tarragon
    1 teaspoon dried thyme

PART II

Recipes

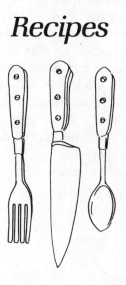

Would you believe lasagna, muffins, flaming bananas, waffles and beef stew can all be prepared low in salt, fat and sugar—and still be delectable? All these favorites—and more—are included in our recipe section. The standards that we follow are simple. There is no salt added to any of our recipes, and we have prepared them using available salt-free products.

Some of the recipes will give you a choice of ingredients; for example, we have tested the muffins made with low-sodium baking powder, but we also tell you how to use the regular kind. Most of our desserts are sweetened with fruits and occasionally with honey; even there we have used much less than traditional instructions call for. Our recipes use ingredients that are naturally low in fat, and we give instructions for fat-free methods of cooking foods that are often sautéed or fried. When we use oils, they are used sparingly for flavor. We also suggest substitutes for traditional high fat ingredients.

We emphasize fresh, seasonal products. You will notice that

our recipes always call for fresh parsley, never dried. Most of the ingredients we use are readily available in supermarkets. For special occasions we sometimes call for a product that is a little out of the ordinary. When that happens we give instructions for where to buy it and how to use it.

Because our recipes are low in fat and sugar, they are also low in calories. Ours is not a book for weight loss, per se, but those who are watching their weight will find they can eat many of our foods with impunity. Persons on restricted-sodium or sugar-free diets will find most of our recipes appropriate for their dietary programs; however, they will still have to calculate their daily intake.

First and Foremost—
Breakfast

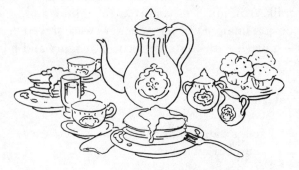

Breakfast customs vary not only from country to country but also from family to family. Some people set the breakfast table the night before; others set out just their reading material. Some people eat standing up, and still others skip breakfast entirely. Weekend breakfasts for many are traditional and leisurely; Sunday brunch is an opportunity to entertain friends.

Whatever your habit has been in the past, begin now to make breakfast a nutritious meal that sets the tone for a day of healthful caring for yourself. In the following chapter we have tried to present some low-fat, low-salt, low-sugar approaches to traditional American breakfast foods—cereals, muffins, waffles, and French toast—as well as some breakfast ideas we brought home from our travels. These foods should fit into any individual's breakfast pattern.

MUESLI

This combination of grains was all the rage in Europe in recent years when high-fiber foods were touted as the best way to lose weight. Now we eat muesli not only for breakfast but as our favorite snack. There are an endless number of foods to combine with it—fresh fruits in season and dried fruits anytime; milk, fruit juices or yogurt as the liquid; and any flavorings you can imagine. In Jerusalem we were served "chocolate soup"—muesli with fresh fruit, cocoa, yogurt and honey.

Basic Muesli Mix

        2 cups oatmeal or rolled oats
        1 cup barley flakes
        1 cup wheat flakes
        1 cup triticale flakes (optional)
        ½ cup unprocessed bran
          cinnamon, to taste

Combine all ingredients and store in airtight container. The quantities may be doubled or tripled.

Makes 5½ cups.

Banana Muesli

        ½ banana
      2–3 tablespoons nonfat or low-fat yogurt
        ½ cup Basic Muesli Mix
        ¼ cup nonfat milk
      1–2 tablespoons raisins
      1–2 tablespoons Grapenuts cereal or toasted wheat
            germ (optional)

In a cereal bowl, mash banana; then mix in yogurt. Stir in muesli. Add milk, raisins and sprinkle with Grapenuts or toasted wheat germ.

Makes one serving.

Orange Juice Muesli

½ cup Basic Muesli Mix
2 tablespoons raisins
½ cup fresh or reconstituted orange juice
2 apples, cored and grated*
1 cup nonfat milk (approximately)

Combine muesli, raisins and orange juice; cover and let sit overnight. In the morning combine muesli mixture with grated apples. Add enough milk to moisten to your taste.

Makes 2 to 3 servings.

Sweet Hot Cereal

We like to prepare this cereal in large quantities and store it. Then on any morning we need only add hot water for a nourishing, tasty breakfast. It's also useful to have on camping trips.

4 cups rolled oats
4–6 tablespoons carob powder
2 teaspoons cinnamon
½ cup instant nonfat dry milk
½ cup raisins

---

*We like the color and texture of apple peels, but if you don't, peel them before coring and grating.

Combine all ingredients. Store at room temperature in a jar or canister with a tight-fitting lid. To prepare hot cereal, combine ½ cup mix with 1 cup boiling water. Simmer for 2 to 3 minutes. Or prepare the cereal the night before and keep it warm in a wide-mouthed Thermos jar.

Makes 2 servings.

Another Granola Recipe

> 2 cups oatmeal
> 1 cup barley flakes
> 1 cup wheat flakes
> ¾ cup orange juice
> 1 teaspoon cinnamon
> 1 teaspoon orange extract

Preheat oven to 350 degrees. Combine grains in a shallow baking pan. Mix together orange juice, cinnamon and extract. Stir juice into grains until they are moistened. Bake for 20 minutes, then stir mixture. Reduce temperature to 300 degrees and continue baking until mixture is brown and crisp, stirring occasionally. Store in an airtight container in the refrigerator.

Makes about 2 cups.

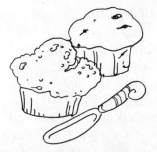

MUFFINS

The sweet, natural flavor of whole grains compensates for their heavier texture. We have used oil in these recipes, but as you become accustomed to their new taste and texture, you may wish to cut out even this small amount of fat.

Basic Muffin Mix

    2 cups rolled oats
    4 cups whole wheat pastry flour, or 2 cups whole wheat flour and 2 cups unbleached white flour
    2 tablespoons baking powder*
    1 tablespoon cinnamon
    1 teaspoon nutmeg
    1 tablespoon dried orange bits (optional)
    1 cup dry buttermilk made from skim milk or 1 cup instant nonfat dry milk

Place oats in blender or food processor and blend until they are the consistency of cornmeal. Pour into a large bowl. Add all remaining ingredients and mix well. Store in airtight container. Bake as instructed in any of the following variations.

---

*If you are using low-sodium baking powder, do not add it to the basic mix; add 4 teaspoons to 2 cups of mix each time you use it.

Blueberry Muffins

2⅓ cups Basic Muffin Mix
1 banana, mashed
1 cup orange juice
1 teaspoon vanilla
2 tablespoons safflower oil
2 egg whites or 1 whole egg
1 cup fresh or frozen blueberries

Preheat oven to 400 degrees. Place mix in a large bowl. In a smaller bowl combine banana, juice, vanilla and oil; mix well. Beat egg whites until stiff; if you are using a whole egg, mix it with the banana and juice. Add banana mixture to muffin mix, stirring just enough to moisten. Add blueberries and stir. Last of all, fold in egg whites. Spoon into nonstick or lightly greased muffin tins and bake for 20 to 25 minutes.

Makes 10 to 12 muffins.

APPLE MUFFINS: Omit blueberries and orange juice from Blueberry Muffin recipe. Replace with ¾ cup grated apple, ¼ cup raisins, 1 cup apple juice or cider, and ¼ teaspoon cinnamon. Makes 10 to 12 muffins.

Pancakes

2 cups Basic Muffin Mix
1 cup water or fruit juice
1 cup nonfat milk
2 egg whites, slightly beaten
1 tablespoon safflower oil

Measure muffin mix into large bowl. In another bowl combine water or juice, milk, egg whites and oil, then pour into muffin mix and stir briefly. Heat nonstick griddle to medium. Pour large spoonfuls of pancake batter onto griddle. Turn pancakes when bubbles appear. Serve with our Grape Jam (p. 57), Uncooked Applesauce (p. 58), Pineapple Cheese (p. 60) or Sweet Tofu Topping (p. 39).

Makes 12 to 15 pancakes.

Bran-Raisin Muffins

Work quickly when you are using low-sodium baking powder. Be certain the oven is preheated and the pans are ready. Low-sodium baking powder begins to react just as soon as it is mixed with liquid ingredients.

>   1 cup whole wheat pastry flour
>   1 cup unprocessed bran
>   1 teaspoon cinnamon
>   4 teaspoons low-sodium baking powder or
>   2 teaspoons regular baking powder
>   1 cup orange juice
>   1 cup raisins
>   2 teaspoons blackstrap molasses
>   ½ teaspoon grated orange rind (optional)
>   2 tablespoons safflower oil
>   2 egg whites, beaten until stiff
>   ¼ cup orange juice (optional)

Preheat oven to 350 degrees. In a large mixing bowl combine flour, bran, cinnamon and baking powder. In a separate bowl mix together orange juice, raisins, molasses, orange rind and oil. Combine liquid ingredients with dry, stirring just enough to moisten. Fold in egg whites. Immediately pour batter into nonstick muffin tins until they are two-thirds full. Bake for 20 to 25 minutes. Brush ¼ cup orange juice on warm muffins if desired.

Makes 10 to 12 muffins.

Overnight French Toast

You will be amazed to see how little fat it takes to "fry" if you heat the frying pan first and then brush a very thin layer of melted margarine onto the pan.

> ¼ cup nonfat milk
> 2 tablespoons instant nonfat dry milk
> 1 teaspoon frozen juice concentrate
> 1 egg white
> ½ teaspoon sesame seeds
> 2 slices whole wheat bread
> ¼ teaspoon unsalted margarine, melted

In a shallow bowl large enough to hold two slices of bread, combine the liquid and dry milks, juice concentrate, egg white and sesame seeds, and mix thoroughly. Lay the bread in the mix and turn once. Cover and refrigerate overnight. The next morning, or when liquid is completely absorbed, preheat a large frying pan to medium. Brush the pan with the margarine. Lay the bread slices in the pan and "fry" them until brown; turn and cook the other side. Serve with our Grape Jam (see p. 57) or Uncooked Applesauce (see p. 58).

Makes one serving. Recipe can easily be expanded.

Eggless Waffles

    1 cup nonfat milk
    1 teaspoon vanilla
    1 tablespoon safflower oil
    2 tablespoons apple juice
    2 tablespoons honey
    2 cups minus 2 tablespoons whole wheat pastry
        flour
    1 teaspoon baking powder or 2 teaspoons low-
        sodium baking powder
    3 tablespoons sesame seeds (optional)

Combine milk, vanilla, oil, juice and honey. Add flour, baking powder and sesame seeds to liquid ingredients. Bake in your waffle iron according to manufacturer's instructions. Serve with applesauce and/or yogurt or our Sweet Tofu Topping (see p. 39). Omit honey and serve unsweetened waffles with chicken or fish in white or Velouté Sauce (see p. 30 and p. 31).
    Makes 2 waffles.

Grape Jam

    This technique will work with any fresh fruit. The jam will keep for up to two weeks in the refrigerator, or it can be frozen if it is made with sweet rice flour. Do not peel your fruits; the skins will cook down and add color and flavor to your jam.

    1 pound sweet red grapes, seeded
    2 tablespoons frozen pear-grape juice concentrate
        or other fruit juice concentrate
    1 tablespoon sweet rice or potato flour

Puree grapes in food processor or blender. In a small sauce-pan combine grapes and juice concentrate. Bring to a boil, stirring constantly. Reduce heat and simmer for 5 minutes. Drain 2 to 3 tablespoons of juice from mixture and set aside to cool. Cook grapes 15 to 20 minutes longer. Stir flour into cooled juice, then add mixture to pan. Simmer jam until thickened.

Makes about 1½ cups.

Uncooked Applesauce

We like the texture and color that apple peel adds. However, you may pare your apples if you prefer to, especially if you can't find unwaxed apples.

> 2 medium apples, cut into chunks
> ¼ cup pineapple juice, no sugar added
> ½ teaspoon cinnamon

Place all the ingredients in a blender or food processor. Blend to desired consistency. Cover and store applesauce in the refrigerator; keeps for up to one week.

Makes about 1 cup.

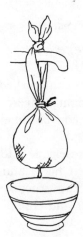

YOGURT CHEESE

Cream cheese is almost entirely fat, while our Yogurt Cheese contains almost no fat and half as much sodium. Use our Yogurt Cheese for traditional brunches with bagels, English muffins or breads and a variety of fruit or fish spreads.

Basic Yogurt Cheese

Line a large strainer or colander with two or three layers of fine cheesecloth. Spoon 2 cups of low-fat or nonfat yogurt into the center of the cloth. Gather the corners of the cloth and pull them up. Twist them together to form the yogurt into a tight ball in the center of the cloth. Fasten with a twist tie or rubber band near the ball. Tie the remaining long ends of cheesecloth to a faucet or cupboard handle so that the "whey" can drip from the cheese. Let the cheese drip out for at least 6 hours or overnight, and be sure you have a dish underneath to catch the liquid. The whey is full of nutrients and can be added to soups, sauces or vegetable dishes. Put the yogurt ball in a strainer with a weight on top to force out even more liquid. (A plastic bag of dry rice or beans makes a good weight.) Press down on the weight occasionally to remove the last bit of whey. Yogurt Cheese is ready when it is the solid consistency of cream cheese.

Pineapple Cheese

> One 8-ounce can crushed pineapple, no sugar added
> 1 cup Yogurt Cheese
> ¼ cup dried fruit, finely chopped

Drain pineapple, reserving 2 to 3 tablespoons juice. Combine pineapple, Yogurt Cheese and reserved juice in a food processor or blender and process until well mixed. Stir in dried fruit. Cover cheese and chill.

Makes about 2 cups.

Fish Spread

For a quick appetizer serve Fish Spread formed into balls and rolled in finely chopped parsley or chives.

> 1 cup Yogurt Cheese
> ½ cup cooked fish, such as salmon
> 2–3 sprigs fresh dill, chopped, or ½ teaspoon dry
> 1–2 tablespoons grated onion

Combine all ingredients and mix well.

If you can "afford" extra sodium, this spread made from smoked fish and Yogurt Cheese is delicious.

Vegetable Frittata

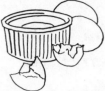

All leftover vegetables needn't go into soup. Some of them can go into a Vegetable Frittata.

1–2 tablespoons unsalted, defatted stock (see pp. 25–28)
1 medium onion, finely chopped
1–2 cloves garlic, minced or mashed
½ teaspoon dry mustard
1 cup finely chopped zucchini
¼ cup sliced mushrooms
½–1 cup additional finely chopped vegetables, either leftovers or any combination of fresh, such as red or green peppers, cooked corn, tomatoes or dried green chili peppers
3 egg whites and 1 egg yolk
¼ cup grated low-sodium or low-fat cheese
3–4 sprigs fresh parsley, finely chopped
freshly ground pepper to taste

Preheat oven to 350 degrees. Heat stock in a large nonstick frying pan. Add onion and cook for 2 to 3 minutes. Add garlic and dry mustard. Cook 1 to 2 minutes more. Add zucchini and mushrooms and continue cooking for 2 to 3 minutes. Add additional fresh vegetables to zucchini mixture; add any cooked vegetables when the others are crisp-tender. Cool.

Meanwhile, beat egg whites and yolk, then add cheese. Remove vegetables from frying pan with slotted spoon and add to egg-cheese mixture. Continue to simmer the vegetable juices remaining in the pan until reduced to 1 tablespoon. Stir concentrated vegetable juices into egg mixture. Add parsley and ground pepper. Pour mixture into 8-inch nonstick pan and bake for 30 minutes or until lightly browned.

Makes 6 servings.

Blueberry Kugel

Serve this traditional noodle pudding for brunch, as the entrée for a light lunch or as dessert after a vegetable meal.

    6–8 ounces wide noodles
      1 cup low-fat cottage cheese
      1 cup Sweet Tofu Topping (see p. 39)
      1 cup crushed pineapple, no sugar added, drained,
           or 1 cup mandarin oranges, no sugar added
      2 cups fresh or frozen blueberries
         toasted wheat germ (optional)

Preheat oven to 350 degrees. Cook noodles according to package directions, omitting the salt. Puree cottage cheese and Sweet Tofu Topping in food processor or blender. Stir in fruits. Add noodles to cheese-fruit mixture. Pour into shallow, lightly greased or nonstick baking dish and bake for 30 minutes. Sprinkle with wheat germ if desired and bake 5 more minutes. Serve hot or at room temperature.

Makes 6 to 8 servings.

Entrées Are Main Dishes

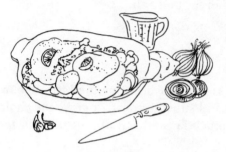

Entrée is a word of unusual history. It comes from the French word *entremets,* which meant the light or sweet dishes served between the heavier courses of a formal meal. As tastes changed and menus became simpler, the word *entrée* came to mean the main dish itself, the focus for the meal and usually its main source of protein.

With meal planners today becoming more and more concerned with light meals and simple, healthy foods, it is more appropriate than ever that the main dish should be an *entrée,* a light dish that is also nutritious, filling and delicious. In our homes a shift has been made from the years when we served red meat six nights a week with an occasional fish or chicken dish, to just the opposite. Now fish, chicken or meatless main dishes are the rule.

Our favorite recipes follow. They include the familiar standbys of every kitchen—lasagna, macaroni and cheese, meat loaf and even roast turkey—plus a number of different ways to cook fish and chicken. Our meatless main dishes follow practices that vegetarians have known for years: certain combinations such as beans and grains or potatoes and dairy products, eaten together, become complete proteins that are just as nutritious as meat. But in case you develop the sinking feeling that you can never eat red meat again, we have included many recipes that allow you to prepare meat so that it will be low in fat and salt.

Lasagna

Lasagna is the perfect recipe to illustrate our techniques of adaptation and substitution. *You* make the choices that determine how much fat and salt are included in the final dish.

    1 pound fresh spinach, or one 10-ounce package frozen spinach
    ½ pound ground meat (see choices following recipe)
    3 cups Tomato Wine Sauce (see p. 33)
    ½ pound mushrooms, chopped
1–2 tablespoons unsalted, defatted stock (see pp. 25–28)
    1 pound skim-milk ricotta cheese, or 2 cups low-fat (2%) cottage cheese, drained, or 2 cups dry-curd cottage cheese cream substitute (see p. 40)
    2 egg whites
    ¼ teaspoon grated nutmeg
    ½ pound lasagna noodles
    1 clove garlic
4–6 ounces shredded low-fat cheese (mozzarella or a similar type)
    2 tablespoons grated Parmesan or sapsago cheese, or 2 tablespoons grated low-sodium cheese

Preheat oven to 350 degrees. Wash fresh spinach; cook for 2 to 3 minutes in a covered saucepan, using only the water that clings to the leaves, until spinach is limp. Drain well and chop. Or defrost frozen spinach and squeeze dry. (Spinach must be absolutely dry.) Set spinach aside.

Brown meat and drain fat. Add tomato sauce. In a separate pan cook mushrooms in stock briefly, then add to tomato sauce. Mix ricotta cheese, egg whites and nutmeg together.

Cook pasta according to package directions, adding the whole clove of garlic to the water instead of salt. Drain. In a 9-by-13-inch shallow baking dish, layer half each of the sauce, pasta, spinach, ricotta cheese and shredded cheese. Repeat layers. Top with grated cheese.

Bake for 30 minutes. Turn oven off and allow lasagna to sit in oven for an additional 30 minutes.

Makes 4 to 6 servings.

Low-Fat, Low-Salt Choices

Use veal or turkey instead of beef.

Use less or no meat and increase the amount of spinach.

Use the lowest fat soft cheese, in place of ricotta.

Use sapsago cheese instead of Parmesan.

Use salt-free cheeses in place of mozzarella, Parmesan or sapsago.

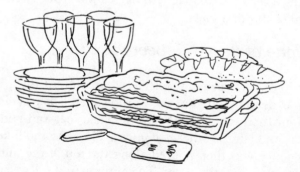

Spaghetti Sauce

> 1 medium onion, finely chopped
> 1–2 cloves garlic, minced
> 1–2 tablespoons unsalted, defatted stock (see pp. 25–28)
> ½ pound ground beef
> One 6-ounce can tomato paste, no salt added
> 2 cups diced fresh tomatoes, or 2 cups canned chopped or stewed tomatoes, no salt added
> ½ cup chopped fresh parsley
> 1 teaspoon oregano
> 2–3 leaves fresh basil, minced, or ½ teaspoon dried
> 1 bay leaf
> ½ teaspoon paprika
> 2 tablespoons apple juice concentrate

In a large frying pan brown the onion and garlic in stock. Remove them from the pan. In the same pan brown the ground beef, breaking up the pieces. Pour off fat and discard. Return onion and garlic to the pan, add tomato paste, tomatoes, seasonings and apple juice concentrate. Cook sauce for about 30 minutes, until thick. Remove bay leaf before pouring over cooked spaghetti or pasta of your choice.

Makes 2½ to 3 cups.

Roulette of Beef with Beet Sauce

Meat loaf is not usually considered an elegant dish, but this one was demonstrated at the Cordon Bleu Cookery School in London. Instructors sliced half the meat loaf and laid it on a platter, and left the other half uncut. The stroganofflike mushroom sauce was then poured along the top of the uncut part and drizzled over the slices. To continue in the Russian style, they served beet relish alongside the meat loaf.

Our version eliminates much of the fat while retaining the flavor. By choosing a good-quality lean beef and mincing it in a food processor, you are assured of extra lean meat. However, you could ask your butcher to mince it for you.

> 1 cup fresh parsley leaves, loosely packed
> 2–3 sprigs fresh thyme, or ¼ teaspoon dried thyme
> 2 shallots or green onions
> 1–1½ pounds top round steak
> 2 tablespoons bread crumbs
> ½ teaspoon dry mustard
> ⅛ teaspoon pepper
> 2 tablespoons cold water
> 1 egg white
> 2–3 green onions, chopped
> ½ pound mushrooms, sliced
> ½ teaspoon paprika
> 2 tablespoons sherry
> 1 cup low-fat or nonfat yogurt
> 1 teaspoon cornstarch or arrowroot
> Beet Sauce (recipe follows)

Preheat oven to 350 degrees. Finely chop parsley and thyme in food processor. Set aside. Chop shallots and set aside. Cut meat into 1-inch cubes, then chop in processor until it resembles hamburger meat. Add chopped herbs, shallots, bread crumbs, mustard, pepper, water and egg white. Process until all ingredients are well mixed. Shape mixture into a roll. Brown the bottom only in a nonstick frying pan. Using a spatula, transfer roll to a loaf pan. Bake for 40 to 45 minutes, basting occasionally with pan juices.

While meat is baking, add onions and mushrooms to the same pan in which the meat was browned. Cook for 3 to 4 minutes, scraping up browned bits from the bottom of the pan. Add paprika and sherry, and cook for 1 to 2 minutes.

Combine yogurt and cornstarch. Stir into onion-mushroom mixture just before serving.

To serve, slice meat; spoon yogurt sauce over and surround with Beet Sauce.

Makes 4 servings.

BEET SAUCE

> 1 pound fresh beets
> 2 teaspoons red wine vinegar
> 1 teaspoon apple juice concentrate
> 1–2 green onions, chopped

Wash beets gently. Cut off all but 1 inch of stem and root. Place in a saucepan and cover with cold water. Bring to a boil. Simmer until beets are tender—about 35 to 50 minutes, depending on size. Skin and mash, then return them to the pan. Stir in remaining ingredients. Cook 2 to 3 minutes more.

Makes about 1 cup.

Meatballs in Sweet and Sour Sauce

These meatballs can be served as a main dish or as an appetizer. If they are part of a supper, serve them with plain steamed rice, either converted white or brown, cooked in water seasoned with a good wine vinegar.

MEATBALLS

> ½ pound ground veal
> ½ pound ground beef
> 1 small onion, finely chopped
> 2 cloves garlic, minced
> 1 teaspoon ground coriander

½ teaspoon ground cumin
¼ teaspoon chili powder
½ teaspoon freshly ground pepper
½ cup soft bread crumbs
¼ cup nonfat or low-fat yogurt

Combine all ingredients in a large bowl. Form mixture into 1-inch balls. Broil balls for 6 to 8 minutes, turning them to brown all over.

Makes about 20 meatballs.

SWEET AND SOUR SAUCE

6–8 small onions, peeled
2–3 carrots, sliced and cut in ½-inch cubes
One 1-pound can pineapple chunks, no sugar added
3 tablespoons tomato sauce, no salt added
1 teaspoon low-sodium soy sauce
¼ teaspoon garlic powder
⅛ teaspoon coriander
1 tablespoon cornstarch, dissolved in 2 tablespoons water
1 green pepper, cut in ½-inch cubes.

Parboil onions and carrots in water to cover for 2 to 3 minutes or until almost tender. Drain and save broth. Drain pineapple, saving juice and adding enough broth to make 1 cup. Combine juice, tomato sauce, soy sauce and seasonings in medium-size saucepan; simmer for 5 minutes. Add cornstarch-water mixture. Stir gently over medium heat until mixture comes to a full boil and sauce thickens. Boil for 1 minute, still stirring; remove from heat. Add onions, carrots, green pepper, pineapple chunks and meatballs. If served as an appetizer, place in a chafing dish, and provide cocktail picks and small plates or napkins for guests. To reheat sauce, cook gently; boiling at this point will cause sauce to thin.

Rolled Flank Steak

A meat roll with a colorful stuffing is part of the cuisine of many countries. While looking for a substitute for the fatty sausage-and-bread stuffings of Europe, we found a recipe for a vegetable-stuffed roll in Latin America. This rolled flank steak, called *matambre,* was developed by the gauchos, Argentinian cowboys, to carry with them as they roamed the Pampas.

Rolling the steaks is a little tricky; it's easier with an assistant, but it can be done by one. We suggest a stuffing of spinach, carrots and leeks for their colors as well as their flavors, but you can substitute any vegetables you like—parsnips or red or green peppers, for example. Just be sure the vegetables are cut into long, narrow strips for easy rolling.

Two 2-pound flank steaks
2 teaspoons finely chopped garlic
½ cup red wine vinegar
3 tablespoons chopped fresh parsley
1 teaspoon salt-free chili powder
1 teaspoon ground cumin
½ teaspoon freshly ground pepper
1 bunch fresh spinach, washed and trimmed (about 3 cups prepared leaves)
2 long fat carrots, scrubbed and quartered lengthwise, or 8 skinny carrots, less than ½ inch in diameter
2 large leeks, washed, trimmed and quartered lengthwise, or 8 green onions
1 large onion, sliced
2 cups dry red wine
1–3 cups unsalted, defatted stock (see pp. 25–28)

Butterfly the steaks in the following manner: using a long, sharp knife, make a horizontal cut through the thickness of each steak from one long side almost but not quite through to the other side. You should have a narrow strip left as a hinge. Open the steaks and, if you wish, pound them flat with a wooden mallet. Lay one steak, cut side up, in a rimmed pan or dish large enough to hold it without folding. Scatter half the garlic and pour half the vinegar over the meat. Lay the second steak, also cut side up, over the first, and dress it in the same way with the remaining garlic and vinegar. Cover with plastic wrap and marinate in the refrigerator overnight or for at least six hours at room temperature.

When you are ready to cook, preheat the oven to 375 degrees. Cut four to five lengths of kitchen twine 2 feet long. Place the steaks on a flat surface, cut side up and end to end. Lay the end of one steak over the other so they overlap by about 2 inches. Pound the overlapped edges with a wooden mallet to join them. Now you should have one long piece of meat with the grain running lengthwise.

In a small bowl mix the parsley, chili powder, cumin and pepper. Scatter these spices over the meat. Make an even layer of spinach leaves over the meat. Lay the carrots and

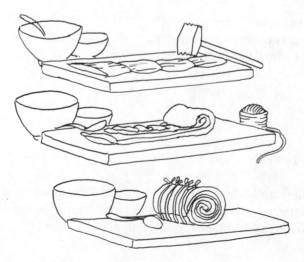

leeks over the spinach across the grain of the meat in a pattern of alternate colors. Arrange the onion slices over the top.

Beginning at one short end, roll the steaks with the grain into a fat cylinder. Slip a length of twine under each end of the cylinder about one inch from the edge and tie the roll securely. Now tie the roll in two or three more places between the first two ties. Lift the roll carefully and place it in a deep casserole or roasting pan just large enough to hold it. Pour in the wine and enough stock or water to bring the liquid a quarter of the way up the side of the roll. Cover tightly and roast in the oven for 1 hour.

Serve the roll hot, removing it from the pan to a cutting board, covering it with foil and letting it sit for 10 minutes first. Or serve it cold, removing it from the pan and chilling it. Cut and remove the strings. Save the pan juices for stock. At the table, cut the roll dramatically into slices and serve.

Makes 10 to 12 servings.

Meat-Filled Dumplings

These versatile dumplings can be the focus of a simple supper, the appetizer of an elaborate dinner or one course in a Chinese meal. Cold dumplings can be carried in a brown-bag lunch or a picnic basket.

DOUGH

> 4 cups flour
> 1½ cups water

Mix flour and water. Add more water a teaspoon at a time until dough cleans bowl. Turn it out on a floured board; knead smooth. Wrap in plastic wrap, and set aside for 20 minutes.

FILLING

> ½ pound ground beef, browned and drained of all
>   fat
> 2 teaspoons low-sodium soy sauce
> 1 teaspoon sherry
> 2 cups fresh spinach, washed, dried and chopped,
>   or 1 cup frozen chopped spinach, thawed and
>   dried
> 1 teaspoon grated fresh ginger
> ¼ cup finely chopped water chestnuts
> 2 green onions, chopped

Combine all ingredients and mix well.

DUMPLINGS

Form dough into a long roll 1 inch in diameter. Cut or break into 1-inch sections. With your hands or a large glass, flatten each piece into a circle 3 inches in diameter. Place 1 tablespoon of filling in the center of each circle. With a finger dipped in water, dampen the edge of the circle. Fold the dough over the filling and press to seal. Brush a nonstick frying pan with ½ teaspoon oil. Place the dumplings in the pan and brown them on each side. Add enough broth or water to come up to a third of the height of the dumplings. Cover pan tightly, and steam until water is all gone—about 15 to 20 minutes. Serve the dumplings hot or cold with sherry or vinegar for dipping.

Marinades for Beef

Picnic main dishes are often grilled hamburgers or meat. If that's your style, choose lean ground beef or flank steak trimmed of all fat, and use one of these marinades for flavor.

BARBEQUE SAUCE

> One 16-ounce can no-salt-added tomatoes
> ½ cup red wine
> ½ cup chopped onion
> 1 carrot, grated
> 1–2 cloves garlic, minced
> 1 tablespoon salt-free chili powder
> ½ teaspoon dry mustard

Drain and chop tomatoes. In a small pan bring all ingredients to a boil; simmer uncovered, stir occasionally, until sauce is slightly thick. Marinate steak in sauce for 3 to 4 hours before grilling; baste hamburgers with marinade while barbecuing.
Makes 1 ½ cups, enough for 2 to 3 pounds of meat.

YOGURT MARINADE

> 1 cup plain low-fat or nonfat yogurt
> 2 tablespoons grated onion
> 2 cloves garlic, mashed or minced
> ½ teaspoon cayenne
> 1 teaspoon turmeric
> ½ teaspoon ginger

Combine all ingredients, then marinate meat for 2 to 3 hours. This marinade is also tasty on chicken (skin removed) or fish.
Makes 1 cup, enough for 1 to 2 pounds of meat.

Chicken Divan

This dish tastes best if the chicken is freshly poached, but for a quick meal, leftovers will do nicely. If you make the sauce with low-sodium cheese, a teaspoon of Worcestershire sauce will add flavor without adding a lot of sodium.

1 pound fresh broccoli
2 tablespoons grated low-fat or low-sodium cheese
2 cups cubed cooked chicken or turkey, skin
    removed
2 cups Velouté Sauce (see p. 30)
¼ teaspoon freshly grated nutmeg
½ teaspoon dry mustard
3 tablespoons sherry
    white pepper to taste
1 teaspoon Worcestershire sauce (optional)
2 tablespoons bread crumbs

Preheat oven to 350 degrees. Cook broccoli by steaming until tender; drain and place in a shallow baking pan. Sprinkle with 1 tablespoon cheese. Arrange chicken on top. Heat Velouté Sauce; add nutmeg, mustard, sherry, pepper and Worcestershire sauce. Pour sauce over chicken and broccoli. Combine remaining cheese with bread crumbs; sprinkle over sauce. Bake for 15 minutes or until hot.

Makes 4 servings.

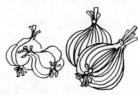

Rosemary Chicken Casserole

2 chicken breasts, split, and 4 thighs
4 medium potatoes, scrubbed and cubed
4 large onions, quartered
½ cup dry white wine
1 tablespoon brandy
1 teaspoon minced fresh rosemary, or ½ teaspoon
    dried
1–2 cloves garlic, minced
1 teaspoon grated orange peel

Preheat oven to 350 degrees. Remove all skin and fat from chicken parts. Brown chicken in a large nonstick skillet, then place it in an oven-to-table baking dish. Add potatoes and onions to skillet and cook in pan juices until lightly browned. Place vegetables in baking dish with chicken. Pour wine into juices in skillet and stir until boiling. Remove pan from heat. Add brandy, rosemary, garlic and orange peel; pour sauce over chicken. Cover dish and bake for 30 minutes or until chicken is tender.

Makes 4 servings.

Chicken Bourguignonne

Small new potatoes are an excellent accompaniment to this traditional French recipe. Steam the potatoes first in a small amount of water. Then brown them in a nonstick pan, using a small amount of Demiglacé Sauce in place of butter.

> 2 tablespoons Unsalted, Defatted Chicken Stock (see p. 26)
> 2 chicken breasts, split, boned and skin removed
> ¾ cup red wine
> 1 tablespoon brandy
> freshly ground pepper to taste
> ½ pound small whole mushrooms, stems removed
> ½ teaspoon margarine, no salt added
> ¾ cup Demiglacé Sauce (see p. 31)

Heat stock in a nonstick frying pan. Add chicken breasts and slowly brown on all sides. Pour wine over chicken. Remove pan from heat. Warm brandy in a small saucepan over low heat; ignite and pour over chicken. When fire has burned itself out, return chicken to heat. Bring sauce to a rapid boil for 1 to 2 minutes. Sprinkle chicken and sauce with pepper. Reduce heat, cover and simmer very gently for 10 to 15 minutes.

While chicken is cooking, cook mushrooms in margarine until slightly golden. Pour Demiglacé Sauce onto chicken and simmer, uncovered, for 2 to 3 minutes more. Place chicken on a hot serving platter. Continue to simmer sauce until reduced by half. Add mushrooms and spoon sauce over chicken.

Makes 4 servings.

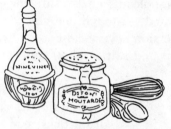

Deviled Chicken

This recipe lends itself to large-quantity cooking. If you plan to prepare chicken for a crowd, broil the pieces briefly just to brown them, and then finish by baking in a moderate oven.

2 tablespoons tarragon vinegar or white wine vinegar
2 tablespoons nonfat or low-fat yogurt
1 tablespoon Dijon-style mustard, no salt added
1 small onion, finely chopped
1 small apple, finely chopped
½ teaspoon ground coriander
½ teaspoon freshly grated ginger
⅛ teaspoon white pepper
1 chicken, cut up and skin removed
chopped tomatoes and minced chives as a garnish

In a small bowl combine all ingredients except chicken and garnish. Score chicken parts with a sharp knife (this allows the marinade to penetrate the meat). Place chicken in a shallow baking pan, cover and marinate overnight in the refrigerator or for 4 hours at room temperature. Remove chicken from marinade and place on broiler pan. Broil until crisp and tender, basting with sauce. Garnish with chopped tomatoes and chives, if desired.

Makes 4 servings.

Chicken Marengo

This classic dish was supposedly invented in the field by Napoleon's chef, using the poor ingredients he had confiscated—a tough, old chicken and some tired vegetables. Our version is very close to the traditional recipe, but without the fat and salt. And, of course, our vegetables are not tired.

2 chicken breasts, skin removed
2 chicken thighs, skin removed
2 drumsticks, skin removed
1 pound small round potatoes, washed and scrubbed
1 medium onion, chopped
2–3 cloves garlic, minced or crushed
2 carrots, sliced
2–3 fresh tomatoes, skin removed and chopped
¼ pound fresh mushrooms, sliced
1–2 tablespoons tomato paste
2 tablespoons whole wheat flour
1½ cups Unsalted, Defatted Chicken Stock (see p. 26)
¼ cup sherry
2–3 sprigs fresh parsley
2 tablespoons chopped fresh basil or ½ teaspoon dried
1 bay leaf
ground pepper to taste

Preheat oven to 350 degrees. Heat a nonstick frying pan and slowly brown chicken pieces on all sides; remove to a casserole. Add potatoes to casserole. In the frying pan, cook onion, garlic and carrots until soft—about 5 minutes. Add tomatoes and mushrooms and continue cooking for 2 to 3 minutes. Stir in tomato paste. Remove pan from heat and stir in flour. Return to burner, and blend in stock. Increase heat until mixture boils, stirring constantly. Add sherry and seasonings. Pour sauce over casserole.

Cover and bake for 1 hour. Remove bay leaf and parsley before serving.

Makes 4 to 6 servings.

Thanksgiving Turkey

Choose a turkey large enough to feed your crowd with some left over for sandwiches. Make sure no salt or fat has been injected into your bird. Avoid the kind that is "self-basting."

Prepare the turkey by first trimming away all the visible fat and excess skin around the body cavity. If you wish, remove most of the skin from the bird's back (the part on the bottom when it lies in the roasting pan).

Rinse the turkey cavity and dry it with paper towels. Do not salt it, and do not rub it with butter or fat. Place a whole orange or an onion, or both, in the cavity to add extra flavor.

Pierce the skin all over with a fork to allow the fat to drain from the bird as it cooks. Place the turkey on a rack in a roasting pan to prevent the bird from cooking in its own fat. Roast it according to standard time and temperature charts. When the bird is finished, transfer it to a heated platter and cover it with foil to keep it warm.

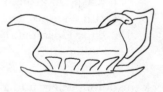

GRAVY

To make gravy, pour the drippings caught in the roasting pan into a fat separator or a jar. Remove fat (see Note p. 26). Measure the broth you have left. Pour the broth into a saucepan and simmer gently. To thicken the gravy, make a paste of

2 tablespoons flour and 4 tablespoons water for each cup of liquid. Stir the paste into the bubbling broth, and simmer until thick. Season to taste with pepper, freshly ground nutmeg, parsley or sage.

For thicker, creamier gravy, add 2 to 3 tablespoons of non-fat dry milk.

STUFFING

Our stuffing roasts alongside the turkey instead of inside and is virtually fat free. Make your own bread cubes from good sourdough or whole wheat bread to avoid the extra salt in commercial stuffing mixes. Of course, those on salt-free diets will choose salt-free bread.

8–10 cups cubed stale bread
   1 medium onion, chopped
   1 cup chopped celery, including the leaves
1–2 cloves garlic, minced
   1 tablespoon safflower oil
8–10 cups cubed stale bread
   ½ teaspoon each sage, thyme, oregano and marjoram, or 2 teaspoons salt-free poultry seasoning
   ¼ teaspoon ground pepper
   ¼ cup chopped fresh parsley
1½ cups Unsalted, Defatted Chicken Stock
       (see p. 26)

Cook the onion, celery and garlic in the oil until soft. Combine all the ingredients in a large bowl and toss lightly. Put the stuffing in a nonstick baking pan and bake, uncovered, alongside the turkey for 1 hour or until top is brown. Cut into squares and serve.

VARIATIONS: Add to the basic stuffing one or more of the following:

> 1 cup chopped fresh mushrooms
> 2 tart apples, chopped
> ½ cup raisins
> 1 cup chopped cooked chestnuts

Baked Whole Fish

Trout and salmon are the fish we most often see whole, but this method of baking can be used with any large fish or piece of fish, such as a "halibut roast." If you have a very large fish, you may want to increase the amounts of stock, mustard and mushrooms.

> One 2–2½-pound fish, cleaned and scaled, or 4 small
>   fish, ½ pound each, cleaned and scaled
> ½ teaspoon onion powder
>   freshly ground white pepper to taste
> 3–4 sprigs fresh dill, or ½ teaspoon dried dill weed
> 3–4 green onions, finely chopped
> 1 tablespoon sherry
> ½ teaspoon Dijon-style mustard
> 3–4 mushrooms, finely chopped
> ½ cup Fish Stock (see p. 28) or dry white wine
> 1 lemon, sliced

Preheat oven to 450 degrees. Season cavity of fish with onion powder and pepper. Tuck dill inside cavity. Place fish on a large piece of foil. If using small fish, place each on a separate piece of foil. Pull up ends of foil so fish sits in middle. In a small bowl combine onions, sherry, mustard, mushrooms and fish stock. Pour mixture over fish; top with slices of lemon. Fold over the edges of the foil and roll them down. The package will look like a canoe with a top. Place package on a rimmed baking sheet and bake for 20 to 25 minutes.

To serve, open package and place fish on a heated serving platter; remove the head and skin, if you wish. Strain the liquid from the foil package into a small saucepan; simmer over low heat until reduced by one-quarter. Pour over fish. Garnish with fresh or dried dill, if desired.

Makes 4 servings.

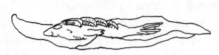

Baked Halibut with Mushroom Sauce

Halibut as we know it is Pacific halibut. It is a firm white fish available fresh on an irregular basis, partly because of the seasonal migration of the fish but also because of limitations on commercial fishing by government agencies protecting the species. Frozen Pacific halibut can be found year-round and is actually more tasty than the so-called Greenland halibut, which is really turbot. Our recipe is best with fresh halibut but will work with any firm white fish steaks.

1½	pounds halibut steaks
½	teaspoon ground coriander
½	teaspoon grated orange rind
2	shallots, finely minced
1	teaspoon margarine, no salt added
½	pound mushrooms, sliced
1	cup low-fat or nonfat yogurt
¼	cup sherry

Preheat oven to 375 degrees. Place halibut in a shallow nonstick baking pan. Sprinkle with coriander and grated orange rind. Using a nonstick pan, cook shallots in margarine. Add mushrooms and cook until soft. With a slotted spoon, remove mushrooms and shallots to a small bowl; add yogurt and sherry. Pour sauce over halibut and bake for 10 to 12 minutes or until fish flakes easily.

Makes 4 servings.

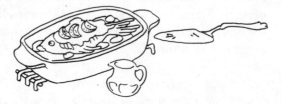

Fish in Wine Sauce

    1   small onion, thinly sliced
1–1½   pounds fish fillets (halibut, snapper, bass)
    1   small tomato, chopped
    ½   cup finely chopped fresh parsley
    1   small red or green pepper, thinly sliced
    ½   cup dry white wine or vermouth
    2   tablespoons lemon juice
    1   tablespoon fresh dill or ½ teaspoon dried
    ¼   teaspoon dry mustard

Preheat oven to 400 degrees. Place onion slices on the bottom of a shallow nonstick baking pan. Place fish on top of onion. Scatter chopped tomato, parsley and pepper over fish. In a small bowl combine wine, lemon juice, dill and mustard. Pour wine mixture over fish. Bake for 15 minutes or until fish flakes easily. Garnish with lemon and dill.

Makes 4 servings.

"Creamy" Hot Crab Casserole

Crabmeat has always been low in fat, but until recently it was considered to be high in cholesterol. Newer research has shown that crab has no more cholesterol, ounce for ounce, than other fish, so we can use it for a scrumptious company casserole.

Sodium is the major problem with shellfish. Fresh-cooked or frozen crab probably has been cooked in salt water, but even so these would be lower in sodium than the canned variety. Fresh crab that you cook yourself is the lowest in sodium; unfortunately fresh crab is available only in a few areas of the country.

2 cups cream substitute (see p. 40)
    2 cups fresh or frozen crabmeat, flaked
    1 small onion, minced
    ½ red or green pepper, finely chopped
  1–2 tablespoons fresh lemon juice
    2 teaspoons horseradish, or to taste
    1 teaspoon Worcestershire sauce
    ½ teaspoon white pepper
One 6-ounce can water chestnuts, drained and finely chopped

Preheat oven to 400 degrees. Blend all ingredients except water chestnuts. Place in a 2-quart casserole; sprinkle with water chestnuts and bake for 10 to 15 minutes. Serve hot with steamed rice.

Makes 8 servings.

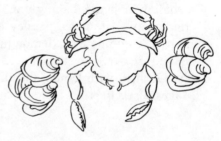

Tuna Noodle Casserole

 ½ cup chopped onion
 ½ cup chopped celery
 1 cup unsalted, defatted stock (see pp. 25–28)
 ½ cup nonfat dry milk
 1 tablespoon flour
 1 tablespoon cornstarch (dissolved in 2 tablespoons water)
 1 tablespoon chopped fresh parsley
 ½ cup shredded or diced low-sodium cheese
 1 teaspoon dry mustard
 1 teaspoon lemon juice
 1 teaspoon dill weed
One 6-ounce can tuna, water packed, no salt added
 6 ounces wide green noodles

Preheat oven to 350 degrees. Cook onion and celery in 1 to 2 tablespoons stock until soft. Remove from heat and sprinkle with milk, flour and cornstarch, and mix well. Return to heat for 2 minutes. Add remaining stock, parsley, cheese, mustard, lemon juice and dill. Drain tuna and add to mixture. Cook for 5 minutes. Meanwhile, cook noodles according to package directions, omitting salt. Drain noodles, then stir into tuna sauce. Place in a nonstick casserole; bake for 25 to 30 minutes.
 Makes 4 servings.

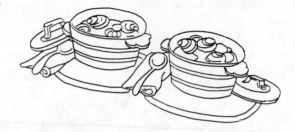

Fish Soup with Clams

1–1½	pounds firm white fish fillets or steaks
15–20	steamer clams in the shell
1–2	tablespoons unsalted, defatted stock (see p. 28)
½	teaspoon olive oil
1	medium onion, finely chopped
1–2	cloves garlic, mashed
½	teaspoon dry mustard
1–2	green onions, finely chopped
½	cup chopped celery
1	medium carrot, thinly sliced
1	small red pepper, sliced
1	teaspoon loosely packed saffron threads
¼–½	teaspoon dried chili pepper
1–2	sprigs fresh thyme, or ½ teaspoon dried
2–3	sprigs fresh parsley, chopped
1	bay leaf
	freshly ground pepper to taste
1	cup dry white wine
3	cups water
1	small potato, diced
1	loaf French bread
1	clove garlic, pressed or pureed

Cut fillets or steaks into 1½-inch cubes and set them aside. Scrub clams. Heat stock and oil in a large soup kettle. Cook chopped onion in stock for 3 to 4 minutes; add garlic and mustard and cook until onions are soft. Add green onions, celery, carrot, red pepper and seasonings. Cook for 2 to 4 minutes. Add wine and water. Bring to a boil, cover and simmer for 5 minutes. Add potato and continue to cook for 15 minutes. Add fish and clams; cook until clams open—about 5 minutes.

Serve hot, topped with toasted French bread that has been rubbed with mashed garlic or garlic puree and browned under the broiler.

Makes 4 servings.

Macaroni and Cheese

Macaroni and cheese has always been a good pantry-shelf meal, a dish that can be prepared quickly from ingredients usually kept on hand. We developed this recipe especially for low-salt diets, using salt-free cheese, but you can substitute low-fat cheese.

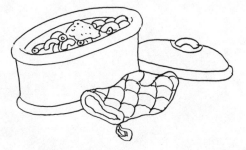

    8 ounces macaroni (made without salt or eggs)
      freshly grated nutmeg
    ½ cup nonfat dry milk
    1 tablespoon flour
    1 tablespoon cornstarch
  One 14½-ounce can stewed tomatoes, no salt added
    ¼ cup chopped onion
    ¼ cup chopped green pepper
    1 cup unsalted, defatted stock (see pp. 25–28)
    8 ounces salt-free Gouda or cheddar cheese or a
      combination, grated
    ¼ teaspoon unsalted margarine (optional)

Preheat oven to 350 degrees. Cook macaroni according to package directions, substituting freshly grated nutmeg for salt; drain and set aside. In a saucepan combine dry milk, flour and cornstarch. Blend in tomatoes, onion and green pepper, and then add stock. Cook, stirring constantly, over medium heat until sauce begins to thicken. Add cheese to sauce. Stir until cheese melts and blends. Add cooked macaroni and freshly grated nutmeg to taste. Bake in a nonstick baking dish or in a casserole lightly greased with unsalted margarine for 30 minutes.

Makes 4 to 6 servings.

Pasta e Fagioli

An Italian tradition: noodles and beans!

> 2 cups dry white beans or pinto beans, soaked
>   overnight
> 4–5 cups water
> 1 teaspoon olive oil
> 1–2 tablespoons unsalted, defatted stock
>   (see pp. 25–28)
> 1 medium onion, finely chopped
> 1 carrot, finely chopped
> 2 cloves garlic, mashed
> ½ teaspoon dry mustard
> ¼ cup grated potato or parsnip (optional)
> 2 tablespoons tomato paste
> 1 teaspoon crumbled oregano leaves
>   freshly ground pepper to taste
> 1 cup orzo (tiny soup pasta)
>   finely chopped fresh parsley (garnish)
> 1–2 tablespoons grated low-fat cheese (optional)

Drain beans; place them in a large soup pot, cover with water and simmer for 45 minutes. Heat oil and 1 tablespoon stock in a small nonstick pan. Add onion and cook for 2 minutes; add carrot and cook 2 minutes more. Add another tablespoon of stock if necessary. Stir in garlic and mustard; cook for 1 minute. Add onion and carrot to beans and cook 45 minutes longer. Add potato or parsnip. Stir in tomato paste, oregano and pepper, and simmer until beans are tender. Cool. Puree half the bean mixture and return it to the pot. Add uncooked pasta and cook for 10 minutes. If mixture seems too thick, add extra stock or a little water or wine. Garnish with parsley and sprinkle with cheese.

Makes 4 to 6 servings.

Beans and Pasta with Artichokes

Artichokes grow like weeds in Italy; we saw bushelfuls of these lovely edible flowers at every market. Alas, unless you grow your own, small artichokes are not available in this country. Our recipe uses frozen artichoke hearts, which do not have the same fresh flavor but still add a distinctive touch to beans and pasta. Avoid canned artichoke hearts; they are usually very salty.

         1 cup pasta shells
         1 clove garlic
         1 cup cream substitute (see p. 40)
     One 14-ounce can no-salt-added whole tomatoes,
           drained and chopped
         1 cup Piquant Tomato Sauce (see p. 32)
       3–4 leaves fresh basil, minced, or ½ teaspoon dried
         ½ teaspoon crumbled leaf oregano
         ½ teaspoon onion powder
         ¼ teaspoon dry mustard
         ⅛ teaspoon freshly ground pepper
       3–4 cloves garlic, mashed
         2 cups cooked pinto or white beans
         1 package frozen artichoke hearts, thawed but
           uncooked
         3 tablespoons grated low-fat or low-sodium cheese

Preheat oven to 350 degrees. Cook pasta as directed in a large pot of boiling water to which you have added 1 whole un-peeled garlic clove instead of salt. Drain pasta and discard garlic. Mix pasta with cream substitute and set aside.

Meanwhile, in a medium-size saucepan, combine tomatoes, tomato sauce, seasonings and mashed garlic. Bring mixture to a boil, reduce heat and simmer for 10 to 15 minutes. Add beans and artichoke hearts to tomato sauce.

Spread half the bean mixture in the bottom of an 8-inch oven-to-table baking dish; top with "creamed" pasta and cover with remaining tomato sauce. Sprinkle with cheese and bake for 30 minutes.

Makes 4 servings.

Bean Curry

>   1 cup small white beans, soaked overnight
>   1 small potato, diced
>   1 clove garlic
>   2½ cups water
>   1–2 tablespoons unsalted, defatted stock
>   (see pp. 25–28)
>   1 large onion, finely chopped
>   ½ cup chopped celery
>   2 cloves garlic, mashed
>   ½ teaspoon freshly grated ginger
>   ¼ teaspoon turmeric
>   ¼ teaspoon finely chopped dried chili peppers
>   ½ teaspoon curry powder
>   ¼ teaspoon cinnamon
>   juice of 1 lemon
>   2 green apples, finely chopped
>   2 cups hot cooked rice

Drain beans; cook beans, potato and unpeeled garlic in water until beans are soft—about 60 minutes. Drain; save cooking liquid but discard garlic. Meanwhile, heat stock in a nonstick frying pan. Cook onion in stock until soft; add celery and mashed garlic. Continue cooking for an additional 2 to 3 minutes. Stir in seasonings and lemon juice, adding extra stock if mixture seems dry. Stir in apples. Add beans, potato and ½ cup cooking liquid to onions, celery and apples; cover and cook for 10 minutes. Serve over hot rice.

Makes 4 servings.

Black Bean Chili

In India spices are frequently roasted or cooked dry to enhance their flavor. We toast our spices in a pan to achieve the same effect.

½ teaspoon cumin seeds
⅛ teaspoon cayenne
½ teaspoon paprika
1–2 tablespoons unsalted, defatted stock (see pp. 25–28)
1 medium onion, chopped
2–3 cloves garlic, minced
1 teaspoon salt-free chili powder
½ teaspoon dry mustard
2 large tomatoes, chopped
¼ cup tomato puree, no salt added
½ green or red pepper, chopped
One 4-ounce can diced green chilies
3 cups cooked black beans
4 ounces shredded low-fat cheese

In a small dry frying pan, toast the cumin seeds over medium heat for 2 to 3 minutes until they begin to pop. Add cayenne and paprika and cook for 1 minute more. Heat stock in a large nonstick frying pan, then add onion and cook for 2 to 3 minutes; add garlic and cook 1 to 2 minutes longer. Combine toasted spices, chili powder, mustard, tomatoes, tomato puree, green or red pepper and chilies. Add this mixture to the onion. Bring to a boil, reduce heat and simmer for 15 minutes. Add cooked beans and continue cooking for 20 minutes. Stir in cheese. Serve warm.

Makes 4 to 5 servings.

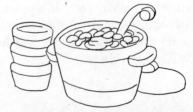

Lentils and Rice, Israeli-Style

In a tiny Moroccan restaurant in Makhane Yehuda, the big open air market in Jerusalem, we were served a delicious dish with an unpronounceable name. We were able to replicate the dish, but not the name, so we call it simply Lentils and Rice, Israeli-Style.

           1 cup dry lentils
           2 cups water
         ½ teaspoon turmeric
         ½ teaspoon grated fresh ginger
       1–2 cloves garlic, minced
         ½ teaspoon dry mustard
           1 cup rice
           2 cups water
           1 tablespoon vinegar
         ¼ teaspoon white pepper
           2 fresh ripe tomatoes
           1 large cucumber
         ½ green pepper
           2 green onions
       1–2 sprigs fresh parsley
           2 large white or yellow onions
           1 tablespoon Vegetable Stock (see p. 27) or more if needed

Rinse the lentils well. Cover with 2 cups water and add turmeric, ginger, garlic and mustard. Bring to a boil and simmer until lentils are soft but still whole—about 20 minutes. Drain and keep warm. At the same time cook the rice with 2 cups water, vinegar and white pepper until all the water is absorbed and the rice is tender.

Meanwhile, prepare a salad in the Israeli style: finely dice the tomatoes, cucumber, green pepper, green onions and parsley. Combine all the diced vegetables and set them aside.

Cut the white or yellow onions into thin slices, then cut the slices in half. Put 1 tablespoon Vegetable Stock in a hot frying pan, add the onions and "fry" until the onions are dark brown. Watch them carefully. Add more broth if the pan becomes dry, but don't add so much that the onions stew; they should be brown.

To serve, spread the hot rice on a platter; heap the hot lentils on top, leaving a border of rice all around. Mound the salad on top of the lentils. Finally, top the salad with the "fried" onions.

Makes 4 hearty servings.

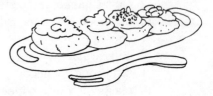

Stuffed Baked Potato

Baking a potato is one of the best ways to preserve its nutrients, especially vitamin C. A medium-size potato baked at 400 degrees will be done in about an hour. However, potatoes will bake at any temperature alongside something else; just allow more time at lower temperatures.

The following recipes will give you several ideas for stuffing potatoes to make them a meal. They all follow this basic format.

1. Wash and scrub potatoes with a vegetable brush.
2. Stab potatoes with a knife once or twice to allow steam to escape while they cook (otherwise potatoes may explode).
3. Bake potatoes until done. A potato should "give" when squeezed. Use an oven mitt when testing.
4. Cut potatoes in half, scoop out the potato pulp and mix with the stuffing.

5. Refill potato shells and serve warm.

6. If potatoes and stuffing are prepared ahead of time, they can be reheated by placing them in a 350-degree oven for 10 to 15 minutes.

HERBED BEEF STUFFING

½ pound lean ground beef, veal or turkey
¼ cup finely chopped celery
1 medium onion, finely chopped
2 cloves garlic, minced
1 tablespoon finely chopped fresh mint, or 1 teaspoon dried
1 teaspoon dried oregano
¼ cup finely chopped fresh parsley
1 cup plain low-fat or nonfat yogurt
4 large potatoes, baked as directed in steps 1–4 chopped fresh tomatoes and cucumber (as garnish)

Brown meat in a frying pan over medium-high heat. Drain all fat. Add celery, onion and garlic to meat and continue cooking until onion is tender. Add seasonings and yogurt and cook over low heat until mixture is heated. Mix with potato pulp from baked potatoes. Garnish with chopped tomatoes and cucumbers, if desired.

Makes 4 servings.

CHEESY POTATO STUFFING

4 large potatoes, baked as directed in steps 1–4
½ cup low-fat cottage cheese
3 tablespoons nonfat milk
2 tablespoons chopped fresh parsley
1 tablespoon fresh lemon juice
¼ teaspoon curry powder

Scoop pulp from potato halves and transfer to a food processor or blender. Add remaining ingredients and mix until smooth. Stuff potato shells with potato-cheese mixture. Return to oven and bake until stuffing is heated—about 10 minutes.

Makes 4 servings.

VARIATIONS: Use ⅛ teaspoon celery seed, ½ teaspoon dried dill weed and 1 teaspoon prepared mustard, no salt added, in place of lemon juice and curry powder.

This basic stuffing is also very good in baked sweet potatoes. When using sweet potatoes, add 1 mashed banana with the cottage cheese.

FLORENTINE STUFFING

    2 cups fresh spinach, or one 10-ounce package
        frozen spinach
    1 cup Basic White Sauce (see p. 29)
  ¼ pound mushrooms, chopped
    2 tablespoons sherry
        freshly grated nutmeg to taste
    4 large potatoes, baked as directed in steps 1–4

Wash fresh spinach; cook for 1 to 2 minutes, drain well; or defrost and drain frozen spinach. (Spinach must be dry.) Chop and mix with warmed white sauce. Cook mushrooms in sherry, and season with nutmeg. Add mushrooms to sauce. Mix potato pulp with spinach sauce and pile back into potato shells. Serve warm.

Makes 4 servings.

Potato-Zucchini Casserole

This basic vegetable recipe is an easy one-dish supper for summertime, when zucchini and fresh basil are plentiful.

1	cup low-fat cottage cheese
¼	cup chopped fresh basil leaves
1	teaspoon crumbled leaf oregano
1–2	cloves garlic, mashed
1–2	tablespoons unsalted, defatted stock (see pp. 25–28)
4	cups sliced zucchini
1	small onion, sliced
2	cups cubed cooked potatoes
2	tablespoons low-fat or low-sodium cheese, grated paprika (as garnish)

Preheat oven to 350 degrees. Mix together cottage cheese, basil, oregano and garlic. Set aside. Heat stock in a large skillet. Add zucchini and onion and cook over high heat until tender-crisp. Remove from heat. Stir in potatoes. Turn zucchini-potato mixture into a 9-inch nonstick baking pan. Spread cottage cheese mixture on top. Sprinkle with grated cheese. Bake uncovered for 20 to 30 minutes or until heated through. Garnish with paprika before serving.

Makes 4 to 6 servings.

Rice-and-Vegetable Casserole

The combination of grains with dairy products increases the amount of available protein in this meatless main dish.

        2¼ cups water
         1 cup long-grain brown rice
        ¼ teaspoon turmeric
         1 teaspoon safflower oil
        ¼ cup Vegetable Stock (see p. 27)
         1 medium onion, sliced
         2 medium leeks, sliced, or 4 green onions, sliced
         2 medium carrots, sliced
         3 medium zucchini, sliced
      4–5 small tomatoes, thickly sliced
         2 tablespoons finely chopped fresh parsley
        ¼ teaspoon marjoram
        ⅛ teaspoon thyme
            freshly ground pepper to taste
         1 tablespoon whole wheat flour
         1 egg white, beaten
        ½ cup low-fat or nonfat yogurt
         1 tablespoon toasted sesame seeds (optional)

Preheat oven to 350 degrees. Bring water to a boil; add rice and turmeric. Reduce heat, cover and simmer for about 40 minutes. Meanwhile, heat oil and 1 tablespoon stock in a large nonstick frying pan. Cook onion and leeks until they begin to brown. Add carrots and 2 tablespoons stock. Cover pan and simmer until carrots begin to soften—about 5 minutes. Stir in zucchini and tomatoes; continue cooking for 5 minutes. Add parsley, marjoram, thyme and pepper. Pour rice into a large casserole; stir in vegetables and remaining stock. Add flour to beaten egg white and beat until smooth. Stir in yogurt. Pour yogurt sauce over rice, and sprinkle on sesame seeds. Cover and bake for 30 minutes.

Makes 4 servings.

Colcannon

Traditionally eaten in Ireland on Halloween or All Hallow's Day, Colcannon should correctly be made with kale, although green cabbage may be substituted. A plain gold ring, a sixpence, a thimble and a button are often put into the mixture to tell the fortune of the diners. The ring means marriage within a year; the sixpence denotes wealth; the thimble, a spinster, and the button, a bachelor, to whoever gets them.

> 3 medium potatoes
> 2 cups fresh kale leaves, washed and stems removed
> ⅓ cup chopped fresh leeks, or ⅓ cup chopped green onions
> 1 cup nonfat milk
> 2 teaspoons unsalted margarine
> freshly ground nutmeg to taste
> freshly ground pepper to taste

Wash and scrub potatoes, then cook them in a small amount of water until soft. Cook kale in a small amount of water until limp; usually the water that clings to the leaves after washing is sufficient. Drain kale well and chop fine. Cook leeks in milk until tender—about 10 minutes; add margarine. Drain potatoes and mash well by hand or electric mixer. Add leeks in warm milk and continue beating. Finally blend in the kale, beating until well mixed. Season to taste with nutmeg and pepper. Serve warm.

Makes 4 servings.

The Jolly Green Grocer— Vegetable Dishes

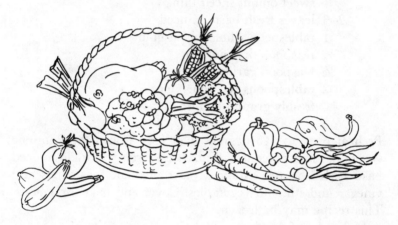

There is nothing better than fresh vegetables, simply prepared or even served raw. Half the produce in our gardens never even makes it to the kitchen. That's why we're not giving you recipes for asparagus or edible pea pods—they're so good just as they are, and so expensive and of such short season, that we never have the opportunity to tire of them. Instead, we are sharing our recipes for those vegetables that are available almost year-round and those that many home gardeners raise in such abundance that their friends are weary of gifts. These recipes are a little more complicated than the steamed or stir-fried methods we all know; many of them are suitable for freezing.

Corn-Zucchini Casserole

        6 ears fresh corn
        6 small zucchini, sliced
        4 medium tomatoes, quartered
      ½ green or red pepper, sliced thin
        1 sweet onion, sliced thin
    2–3 leaves fresh basil, minced
        1 tablespoon whole wheat flour
      ½ teaspoon dry mustard
      ½ teaspoon garlic powder
        2 tablespoons red wine vinegar
          freshly ground pepper to taste

Preheat oven to 325 degrees. Cut corn from cob. Combine vegetables and place in a 2-quart casserole. Sprinkle minced basil leaves on top. Make a paste of flour, seasonings and vinegar and stir into vegetables. Cover and bake for 1 hour. This recipe may be frozen.

Makes 4 to 6 servings.

Tangy Green Beans

    1½ pounds fresh green beans
      ¼ cup unsalted, defatted stock (see pp. 25–28)
        2 cloves garlic, minced
      ¼ teaspoon dry mustard
        1 tablespoon whole wheat flour
        1 tablespoon balsamic vinegar
        1 cup boiling unsalted, defatted stock or water (see
          pp. 25–28)
          finely chopped water chestnuts (optional)

Wash beans and cut into 1-inch lengths. Heat the ¼ cup stock in a large nonstick frying pan. Add the beans, garlic and mustard. Bring to a boil, cover, reduce to low heat and simmer for 6 to 8 minutes. Remove lid and sprinkle flour over beans. Add vinegar and boiling stock. Continue cooking, uncovered, until beans are tender-crisp. Garnish with water chestnuts, if desired.

Makes 4 servings.

VARIATION: Add 1 to 2 small carrots, sliced thin, along with the beans.

Green Beans with Green Grapes

    1 pound fresh green beans
    1 cup seedless green grapes
       juice of half a lemon or lime
       grated rind of half a lemon or lime
   ½ cup unsalted, defatted stock (see pp. 25–28) or water
   ⅛ teaspoon coriander
   ⅛ teaspoon freshly grated nutmeg

Wash beans, snap off ends and break into 2-inch lengths. Place in a medium-size saucepan; add grapes, lemon or lime juice and rind, stock or water, and seasonings. Bring to a boil, cover, reduce heat and simmer for 10 minutes or until beans are tender-crisp. Remove beans to a serving dish. Cook remaining liquid rapidly for 2 to 3 minutes. Pour sauce over beans.

Makes 4 servings.

Cabbage, Onions and Tomatoes

1	cup plus 1 tablespoon unsalted, defatted stock (see pp. 25–28)
1	medium green cabbage, sliced thin
1	medium yellow onion, sliced thin
2	large tomatoes, coarsely chopped
1	tablespoon Dijon-style mustard, no salt added
2	tablespoons whole wheat flour
1	teaspoon poppy seeds (optional)
¼	cup finely chopped fresh parsley
	freshly ground pepper to taste
3–4	tablespoons low-fat or nonfat yogurt

Preheat oven to 350 degrees. Pour ½ cup stock into a shallow range-to-oven baking pan. Stir cabbage into stock; bring to a boil over high heat. Cover and place in oven. Heat 1 tablespoon stock in a medium-size nonstick frying pan. Cook onion until soft. Scatter over cabbage and return baking pan to oven. Add tomatoes to frying pan. Stir in mustard, flour, remaining stock, poppy seeds, parsley and pepper. Bring to a boil and cook for 5 minutes. Spoon tomatoes over cabbage. Bake covered for 45 to 60 minutes, basting occasionally, until cabbage is tender. Stir in yogurt and heat until warm.

Makes 4 to 6 servings.

Seasoned Broccoli

>   1 pound fresh broccoli
>   ⅔ cup unsalted, defatted stock (see pp. 25–28)
>   1 large onion, chopped
>   1–2 cloves garlic, mashed
>   2 medium tomatoes, diced
>   2–3 leaves fresh basil, or ½ teaspoon dried
>   2 tablespoons finely chopped fresh parsley
>   freshly ground pepper to taste

Wash broccoli; slice stems on the diagonal and separate flowerets. Set aside. Heat 1 tablespoon stock in a large non-stick frying pan. Add onion and cook until soft—about 3 minutes; add garlic and cook 1 to 2 minutes longer. Stir in tomatoes and remaining stock. Bring to a boil, then reduce heat and simmer for 3 to 5 minutes. Add broccoli, basil, parsley and pepper. Cover and simmer until tender-crisp. Place broccoli in a serving bowl. Cook remaining sauce until it is reduced by half. Pour sauce over broccoli.

Makes 4 servings.

Leeks with Mushrooms and Tomatoes

Just a small amount of olive oil is enough to give your foods extra flavor, especially if your stock is weak.

>   4 medium leeks
>   1–2 tablespoons unsalted, defatted stock
>   (see pp. 25–28)
>   ½ teaspoon olive oil
>   2 tablespoons chopped fresh parsley
>   ¼ pound small whole mushrooms
>   1 tomato, finely chopped

½ teaspoon freshly grated ginger
¼ teaspoon ground coriander
freshly ground black pepper

Wash leeks, cut off root ends and tough green tops; slice into 1-inch lengths. You should have 2 to 2½ cups sliced leeks. Heat stock and oil in a large nonstick frying pan. Add leeks and cook until soft—about 5 minutes. Sprinkle with parsley; add mushrooms, tomato and seasonings. Turn up heat and stir briskly for 1 to 2 minutes. Cover, reduce heat and cook 2 to 3 minutes longer.

Makes 4 servings.

Corn Kabob

If you have abandoned corn on the cob because you can't imagine eating an ear of corn that doesn't drip butter and salt, don't despair. Our grilled corn leaves the fingers just as messy and delicious to lick as we remember from our childhood.

½ cup low-fat or nonfat yogurt
1 teaspoon garam masala*
1 medium onion, finely chopped
½ teaspoon chili powder
4 ears fresh corn

Beat yogurt with a fork until creamy. Mix in spices and onion. Spread mixture on corn and wrap in foil. Place on a grill until tender—about 15 to 20 minutes. Or pull back corn husks, spread on yogurt mixture, replace husks and grill.

Makes 4 servings.

*Garam masala is a combination of spices from India, available in many spice shops or specialty food stores. It contains black pepper, cardamom, cinnamon, cloves, coriander and cumin.

Spaghetti Squash

Spaghetti squash is fun to serve. Since the cooked pulp resembles strands of spaghetti, it can be used instead of rice or pasta for stir-fry vegetables or any of your favorite pasta sauces. Cut the cooked squash in half and discard the seeds. Then, with a fork, pull out the strands of "spaghetti" and toss with the topping of your choice. Children will especially enjoy the show if you prepare the squash at the table.

> 1 small (2-pound) spaghetti squash
> 1–2 tablespoons unsalted, defatted stock
>   (see pp. 25–28)
> 1 cup coarsely chopped mushrooms
> 1 small zucchini, grated
> 1–2 cloves garlic, mashed
> ½ teaspoon dry mustard
> 1 cup Piquant Tomato Sauce (see p. 32)
> 2 fresh basil leaves, minced, or ½ teaspoon dried
>   freshly ground pepper to taste
> ¼ cup grated low-fat or low-sodium cheese

Preheat oven to 400 degrees. Stab the whole squash once or twice to allow steam to escape during cooking. Place on a

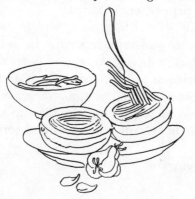

baking sheet and bake until squash "gives" when squeezed. This usually takes 1 to 1½ hours but depends on the size of the squash. Cut the squash in half, discard the seeds and place the "spaghetti" in a large bowl.

Heat 1 tablespoon stock in a large nonstick frying pan. Add mushrooms and cook for 2 to 3 minutes until mushrooms begin to brown; add zucchini. Stir in garlic and mustard. Simmer 3 to 4 minutes. Stir in tomato sauce and simmer 15 minutes more. Add basil and pepper. Pour sauce over "spaghetti." Sprinkle with cheese.

Makes 4 servings.

Marinated Red Peppers and Mushrooms

    1   pound small fresh mushrooms
    ½   cup Unsalted, Defatted Chicken Stock (see p. 26)
    1   tablespoon olive oil
    2   tablespoons sherry vinegar
    1–2 cloves garlic, minced or mashed
    2–3 whole peppercorns
    ½   teaspoon dried oregano
         freshly ground pepper to taste
    1   red pepper, cut in strips

Wash mushrooms and remove stems. In a small saucepan combine the stock, oil, vinegar, garlic, peppercorns, oregano and pepper. Bring to a boil, reduce heat and simmer for 5 minutes. Combine mushrooms and red pepper in a large jar; pour marinade over vegetables and allow to stand for 6 to 8 hours or overnight. Drain vegetables and serve on a bed of salad greens.

Makes 4 servings.

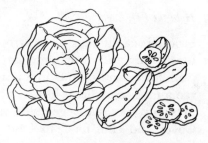

Marinated Vegetables

Marinated vegetables seem to be the "in" food at the trendy take-outs that are opening all over the country. However, low-calorie vegetables become a very fattening dish when the marinade turns out to be mostly oil. Our well-flavored marinade substitutes stock for much of the oil. We suggest some vegetables here, but the marinade works equally well with red or green pepper strips, zucchini slices, mushrooms or brussels sprouts. Leftovers of this salad are delicious over pasta.

1–1½ pounds broccoli*
  1 small head cauliflower
2–3 carrots, sliced thin
  1 red onion, sliced thin and separated into rings
  2 tablespoons safflower oil, or 1 tablespoon olive
     oil and 1 tablespoon safflower oil
  2 tablespoons Unsalted, Defatted Chicken Stock
     (see p. 26)
  3 tablespoons rice wine vinegar
  1 tablespoon Dijon-style mustard, no salt added
2–3 fresh basil leaves
  2 cloves garlic, mashed
     freshly ground black pepper

Wash vegetables. Slice broccoli stems on the diagonal; separate flowerets into small pieces. Break up cauliflower. Blanch

---

* Broccoli will lose its green color in vinegar-based dressings, so it should be added no more than 30 minutes before serving.

broccoli, cauliflower and carrots in boiling water for 2 minutes. Drain and rinse immediately under ice cold water. Place cauliflower and carrots in a large bowl; add onion. Combine remaining ingredients in a jar or a small bowl. Mix well. Pour dressing over all vegetables except broccoli. Toss lightly. Cover and chill for 3 to 4 hours. Add broccoli 30 minutes before serving.

Makes 6 servings.

Summer Potato Garden Salad

It's summertime, and everyone's thoughts immediately turn to picnics. Potato salad, the universal picnic favorite, is often avoided because traditional recipes call for mayonnaise and hard-boiled eggs, and chic gourmet recipes use sour cream and salt. Our colorful salad looks like a creation from a gourmet deli. No one will guess that the fat and salt have been reduced.

    1 cup fresh or frozen peas
    2 green apples, cored and diced but not peeled
    2 small red potatoes, cooked and sliced, not peeled
    1 cup Tofu Mayonnaise (see p. 36) or 1 cup low-fat or nonfat plain yogurt
2–3 teaspoons prepared horseradish (amount depends on strength)
    1 tablespoon chopped fresh mint, or ½ teaspoon dried

Cook fresh peas. Frozen peas may be thawed and added directly to the salad. Mix together apples, potatoes and peas. In a small bowl combine mayonnaise, horseradish and mint. Add dressing to potato mixture and toss gently but well.

Cover and chill for several hours. This recipe is easily doubled.

Makes 4 servings.

Fresh Spinach-Orange Salad

In winter when lettuce is either very expensive or of poor quality, this salad is a welcome change. It always receives rave reviews in our cooking classes.

¼ cup fresh lemon juice
½ cup fresh orange juice
½ teaspoon paprika
1 teaspoon garlic powder
⅛ teaspoon white pepper
1 bunch fresh spinach leaves (about 1 pound)
½ cup sliced turnips or jicama
2 oranges, peeled and cut into bite-size pieces
1 small red onion, thinly sliced

In a small jar or blender, combine juices, paprika, garlic powder and pepper; shake or blend until mixed. Cover and refrigerate until ready to use. Wash spinach and tear into bite-size pieces. Combine with prepared turnips or jicama, oranges and onion in a large salad bowl. Pour dressing over and toss.

Makes 4 servings.

Israeli Eggplant Salad

1 large eggplant
1 teaspoon olive oil or sesame oil

1 tablespoon lemon juice
1 tablespoon grated onion
1 tablespoon dry white wine or vermouth
1–2 cloves garlic, mashed
1 cup low-fat or nonfat yogurt
1–2 fresh mint leaves, minced, or ¼ teaspoon dried
    mint
    red leaf lettuce, red onion, sliced thin, or cherry
        tomatoes and 1 teaspoon sesame seeds as a
        garnish

Preheat oven to 400 degrees. Stab eggplant several times to allow steam to escape, and place on a nonstick baking sheet. Bake until soft—about 45 minutes. Remove from oven and cool; scoop out pulp and chop. Combine pulp with remaining ingredients. Cover and chill several hours or overnight.

To serve, line a platter with red leaf lettuce. Mound eggplant in center, surround with red onion slices or cherry tomatoes and sprinkle sesame seeds over the top.

Makes 4 servings.

Fruit and Cabbage Slaw

½ cup chopped dried apricots
¼ cup raisins or currants
½ cup fresh orange juice
1 medium apple, chopped
1 small cabbage, shredded
1 cup chopped celery
  juice of ½ lemon, approximately 1½ tablespoons

Soak the dried apricots and raisins or currants in the orange juice until the apricots are soft—about 30 minutes. In a large bowl combine apple, cabbage and celery. Add lemon juice and dried fruit mixture. Toss well. Cover and chill 4 hours or overnight. Stir occasionally.

Makes 6 servings.

Ginger Pea Salad

　½　cup low-fat or nonfat yogurt
　½　teaspoon grated ginger
　¼　teaspoon garlic powder
　¼　teaspoon dry mustard
　1　teaspoon low-sodium soy sauce
　1　can water chestnuts, finely chopped
　½　cup grated carrot
　½　cup chopped green onion, including tops
One　10-ounce package frozen peas, thawed, or 1 cup fresh, shelled peas, blanched
1–2　large shredded wheat biscuits, crumbled

Toss together all the ingredients except the wheat biscuits. Refrigerate for at least one hour to allow flavors to blend. Add shredded wheat just before serving.

Makes 6 to 8 servings.

Low-Fat, Salt-Free Caponata

Caponata is a traditional Italian dish served as part of an antipasto. A food processor is a useful tool in this recipe for making all the vegetable slices the same size.

    1 small zucchini, sliced thin
    1 small eggplant, sliced thin
  6–8 mushrooms, sliced thin
    1 medium onion, sliced thin
    2 medium tomatoes, chopped
    1 teaspoon safflower oil
    1 tablespoon sherry vinegar
  1–2 cloves garlic, mashed
    ½ teaspoon dry mustard
    2 sprigs fresh thyme, minced, or ¼ teaspoon dried
    ¼ cup chopped fresh parsley
       freshly ground pepper to taste

Preheat oven to 400 degrees. Arrange vegetables in layers in a shallow 9-by-13-inch baking dish with tomatoes on top. Combine remaining ingredients and pour mixture over vegetables. Cover tightly with foil and bake for 30 minutes. Uncover, lower heat to 300 degrees and continue cooking another 30 minutes or until vegetables are soft. Drain liquid from baking dish, pour into small pan and boil rapidly until reduced by half. Pour over vegetables. Serve at room temperature as part of antipasto or hot over rice, potatoes or pasta.

Makes 4 to 6 servings.

Turnip Relish

In his book *Food* Waverly Root, the famous food historian, said, "Contempt for the turnip as a lowly vegetable reaches far back." For many centuries turnips were food for peasants. In our own time the popular comic strip Li'l Abner featured a hillbilly character who had an uncontrollable passion for "presarved turnips." The humor in this lies in the fact that most of us find turnips bitter and unpleasant. But fresh turnips or those properly stored are less likely to turn bitter, and they are a change from the ordinary in mid-winter. We brought this recipe back from Israel, close to ancient Babylon, where the cultivation of turnips was first recorded.

> 4 turnips, grated (about 2 cups)
> 2 tablespoons fresh lemon juice
> ¼ teaspoon cayenne
> ¼ teaspoon cumin

Combine all ingredients and let stand at room temperature for at least three hours.

Makes 2 cups relish.

VARIATION: Substitute zucchini or jicama for the turnips; use chili powder as seasoning.

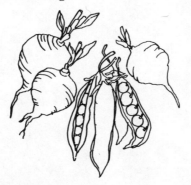

Cranberry-Orange Sauce

This recipe makes a tart sauce. If you wish a sweeter taste, you can add sugar or honey, a spoonful at a time, until it is to your liking. Commercial cranberry sauce contains 80 to 90 percent sugar. With our recipe, you control the amount of sugar you eat.

One	12-ounce package fresh or frozen cranberries
One	12-ounce can frozen orange juice concentrate
¾–1	cup water
2	sweet oranges, peeled, cut into small pieces and seeded
	grated orange rind (optional)

Rinse cranberries under running water. In a medium-size saucepan combine cranberries, orange juice concentrate and water. Stir over medium heat until cranberries pop. Add chopped oranges and rind; cook 3 to 5 minutes longer.

Makes 2½ to 3 cups.

Starches
Don't Need Butter

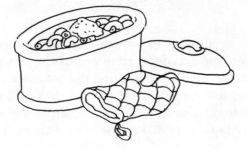

Rich sauces, a pat of butter, a dollop of sour cream—all these give pasta, potatoes and grains an unfair reputation as fattening foods. These starches are actually complex carbohydrates, the chemical name for a combination of carbon, hydrogen and oxygen. Carbohydrates supply glucose, the main fuel needed to run our bodies, and also vitamins, minerals and fiber. They contain the same amount of calories per gram of food as protein (4 calories per gram) and half as much fat (9 calories per gram). A small baked potato contains 90 calories; the pat of butter on top contains more than 100.

When you know it is the *additions* to the starches that make them fattening, you can subtract those rich extras and substitute our low-fat, low-salt sauces and "creams." Use the recipes that follow as models for converting your own favorites.

PASTA

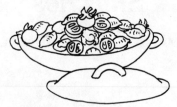

Marco Polo is said to have brought pasta from China to Venice. Within a few decades it transformed the eating habits of the Italians. Originally pasta sauces did not contain tomatoes, for they had not then been introduced as a food in Europe. Nowadays trendy cooks are once again using other than tomato-based sauces to make their pasta dishes appealing and exciting.

HINTS FOR COOKING PASTA

Flavor the cooking water for pasta with garlic, onion or a pinch of the seasonings you will be using in your sauce.

To rewarm cooked pasta, plunge cold noodles into a pan of boiling water for 1 to 2 minutes. Drain immediately.

To separate drained pasta that is stuck together, plunge into cold water, stir, drain and toss with hot sauce.

Mix leftover vegetables into hot pasta sauce.

Use one of our salad dressings (see pp. 34–39) or mix one of our marinated salads (see pp. 108–110) with leftover cooked pasta to make a pasta salad.

Pasta with Primavera Sauce

¼–½ cup defatted, unsalted stock (see pp. 25–28)
1–2 cloves garlic, mashed
½ teaspoon dry mustard
1 medium carrot, sliced thin
2 cups broccoli florets
1 small red pepper, sliced thin
¼ teaspoon ground coriander
freshly ground pepper to taste
1 cup ricotta "cream" (see p. 40)
1 pound pasta, cooked and drained

Heat 1 tablespoon stock in a large nonstick frying pan. Add garlic and mustard; cook for 1 minute; do not brown. Add 1 tablespoon additional stock and the carrot; cook 3 to 5 minutes more. Add remaining stock, broccoli and red pepper. Cook until vegetables are tender-crisp—about 5 to 7 minutes. Add coriander and pepper. Stir in "cream" and heat until sauce is warm. Toss with pasta.

Makes 4 servings.

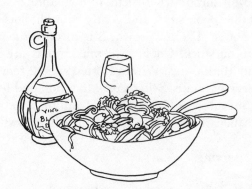

Mushroom Sauce for Pasta

Fresh mushrooms and fresh parsley simmered in a well-seasoned broth provide a welcome change to the traditional tomato-based pasta sauce. If you are fortunate enough to have access to wild mushrooms, the dish will be irresistible.

NOTE: *Never* let mushrooms sit in water. Rinse briefly under the tap and dry gently. If mushrooms absorb water, they lose flavor.

```
  1  pound mushrooms, sliced
  2  tablespoons lemon juice
  1  teaspoon safflower oil
 ¼   cup Unsalted, Defatted Chicken Stock (see p. 26)
  3  small shallots, finely chopped
2–3  cloves garlic, finely chopped
 ½   cup chopped fresh parsley
     freshly ground pepper to taste
     freshly ground nutmeg to taste
     red pepper (as garnish)
  1  pound pasta, cooked and drained
```

Toss sliced mushrooms with lemon juice and set aside. Heat oil and 1 tablespoon stock and gently cook shallots and garlic until they soften. Do not brown. Stir in mushrooms, parsley and remaining stock. Cook until mushrooms are moist and soft—about 10 minutes. With a slotted spoon, remove mushrooms to serving plate. Bring sauce to a boil and heat briskly for 2 to 3 minutes. Add pepper and nutmeg. Return mushrooms to sauce. Toss with pasta. Garnish with strips of red pepper.

Makes 4 servings.

VARIATION: Add 2 tablespoons Madeira or sherry to sauce.

Mushroom, Tomato and Orange Sauce

    1   pound small whole mushrooms (see Note p. 120)
        juice of ¼ lemon, approximately 1 teaspoon
    1   tablespoon olive oil
    ½   cup defatted, unsalted stock (see pp. 25–28)
    1   pound tomatoes, chopped
  2–3   cloves garlic, mashed or finely minced
    1   bay leaf
    2   sprigs fresh parsley
    2   sprigs fresh thyme, leaves only (if fresh thyme is
          not available, omit; do not substitute dried)
        grated rind of ½ orange
        juice of 1 orange
        freshly ground nutmeg to taste
        freshly ground pepper to taste
    1   pound pasta, cooked and drained

Wash and dry the mushrooms. Sprinkle lemon juice on mushrooms and set aside. Combine remaining ingredients except pepper, nutmeg and pasta in a medium saucepan. Bring to a boil, reduce heat and simmer for 10 to 15 minutes. Add mushrooms and cook 3 minutes more. Add pepper and nutmeg. Toss with pasta.

Makes 4 servings.

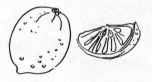

Salmon Pasta Sauce

    1 cup Court Bouillon (recipe follows)
    ½ pound fresh salmon, or 1 cup canned salmon, no
         salt added
    1 cup nonfat Yogurt Cheese (see p. 59)
2–3 sprigs fresh dill, minced, or 1 tablespoon dried
         dill
    1 tablespoon grated onion
2–3 drops Tabasco
    1 pound green pasta, cooked and drained

Bring Court Bouillon to a boil. Add fresh fish and poach for 10 to 15 minutes. Remove salmon, strain broth and cool, or drain canned salmon. Save liquid from either. Flake salmon, discarding any bones and bits of skin. In a small bowl beat the Yogurt Cheese lightly with a fork. Slowly add 2 to 3 tablespoons liquid drained from fish until mixture is the consistency of heavy cream. Mix in salmon. Let mixture sit for 1 hour. Add dill, onion and Tabasco. Serve at room temperature over hot green pasta.

Makes 4 servings.

COURT BOUILLON

    ½ cup white wine
    ½ cup water
    ½ bay leaf
    ½ small onion, cut up
    1 fresh parsley stem
    1 sprig fresh thyme, or ⅛ teaspoon dried
4–5 whole peppercorns

In a small nonstick pan combine all ingredients. Bring to a boil and simmer for 5 minutes.

Makes 1 cup of bouillon.

Linguine with Clam Sauce

Add any extra clam juice you have to the water in which the pasta cooks to flavor the noodles.

         ¼ cup finely chopped onion
         2 shallots, finely chopped
         1 bay leaf
       1–2 parsley stems
         1 sprig fresh thyme, or ¼ teaspoon dried
       4–5 peppercorns
         1 cup white wine
         3 quarts steamer clams (about 24 to 30 clams),
              scrubbed clean
         1 tablespoon olive oil
       2–3 garlic cloves, minced
         ¼ teaspoon dry mustard
         ½ cup finely chopped parsley leaves
            dash red pepper flakes (optional)
         1 pound linguine, cooked and drained

Combine onion, shallots, bay leaf, parsley stems, thyme, peppercorns and wine. Bring to a boil. Add clams and steam for 4 to 5 minutes or until clams open. Remove clams, discarding any that haven't opened, separate them from shells and chop coarsely. Strain and save liquid. Heat olive oil and 1 tablespoon reserved clam juice in a medium-size nonstick frying pan. Add garlic and mustard and cook for 1 minute. Add parsley and cook 1 to 3 minutes more. Add 1 cup reserved clam juice and simmer for 5 minutes or until sauce is reduced by half. Add chopped clams and cook for 1 to 2 minutes. Toss clam sauce with linguine, garnish with lemon, if desired, and serve warm.

Makes 4 servings.

THE POTATO

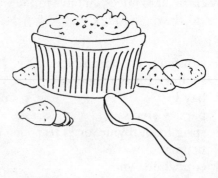

In this country the potato has had a bad press. In France it is the most important vegetable in the cuisine, and a shopper in Manila will buy potatoes to show how affluent he is. Furthermore, the potato not only saved Europe from starvation in the eighteenth century, but because it was easily stored and yielded large crops per acre, it paved the way for the Industrial Revolution. And yet in United States homes and restaurants the potato is fried, dried, shredded, granulated, flaked and frozen, loaded with salt and fat, and then condemned for being fattening and boring.

Properly prepared, the unprocessed potato is a delicious, naturally nutritious source of vitamins, minerals and proteins, one of those rare foods that not only tastes good but is good for you.

Potatoes with Mustard Sauce

        3 medium potatoes
     1½ cups defatted, unsalted stock (see pp. 25–28)
        1 medium onion, chopped
     1–2 cloves garlic, minced
        ½ teaspoon dry mustard
        2 tablespoons whole wheat flour
        2 tablespoons balsamic vinegar
        2 tablespoons low-sodium Dijon-style mustard
        ¼ cup chopped fresh dill, or 2 teaspoons dried
        ¼ cup bread crumbs
           freshly ground pepper to taste

Preheat oven to 350 degrees. Cook potatoes in boiling water to cover until tender; drain and cut into ½-inch slices. In a large nonstick frying pan, cook onion and garlic in 1 tablespoon stock until soft. Stir dry mustard and flour into mixture and continue cooking until color is light brown. Add the remaining stock and the vinegar and stir until boiling. Lower heat and simmer sauce uncovered for 10 minutes. Add Dijon mustard and dill and mix well. Arrange sliced potatoes in a 9-inch nonstick baking pan. Pour sauce over the potatoes. Sprinkle with bread crumbs and bake for 15 minutes.

Makes 4 servings.

Potato Kugel

      2 pounds potatoes, grated
      1 medium onion, grated
      4 tablespoons matzo meal or Roman meal
      ½ teaspoon dry mustard
      1 tablespoon finely chopped parsley
      ⅛ teaspoon pepper
      2 teaspoons low-sodium baking powder, or
            1 teaspoon regular baking powder
      4 egg whites, stiffly beaten
      ½ teaspoon safflower oil

Preheat oven to 375 degrees. Combine potatoes and onion.
Mix together matzo or Roman meal, mustard, parsley, pepper
and baking powder; stir into potatoes. Fold in egg whites.
Pour mixture into a nonstick 8-by-12-inch shallow casserole
that has been brushed with oil. Bake for 45 minutes or until
top is brown.
   Makes 8 servings.

Baked Potato Skins

         baked potatoes
         safflower oil
         seasoning mix (see pp. 41–43)

Preheat oven to 475 degrees. Cut the baked potatoes in half.
Scoop out the inside, leaving ¼- to ½-inch-thick shells. (Save
the potato for soup or other use.) Place skins on a nonstick
pan, cut side down. Use a pastry brush to coat them lightly
with oil. Be a miser; use no more than ¼ teaspoon oil per

potato half. Sprinkle with seasoning mix or any combination of spices. Place in oven for 15 minutes or until potatoes are brown. Allow 1 potato per person.

Potato-and-Lentil Stew

Delicious as a main dish, this stew is also good warmed over or packed for lunch in a wide-mouth Thermos. Therefore we are giving proportions for eight servings, so there will be plenty of leftovers.

```
     1  medium onion, chopped
   2-3  cloves garlic, minced
     2  tablespoons defatted, unsalted stock
          (see pp. 25-28)
   1-2  teaspoons curry powder
     2  cups water
     2  cups dried lentils, washed
     3  medium potatoes, scrubbed and diced
     1  tomato, diced
     2  cups nonfat milk
          juice of ½ lime, approximately 1½ tablespoons
          (optional)
```

In a large soup pot cook onion and garlic in stock until soft—about 5 minutes. Add curry powder, water and lentils. Bring to a boil, cover, reduce heat and simmer for 15 to 20 minutes. Add potatoes, tomato and milk; cover and continue cooking until potatoes are tender. Add lime juice, if desired, and serve warm.

Makes 8 servings.

Potatoes with Onion and Garlic

These potatoes may be assembled early the day they are to
be served and set aside for later baking.

        3 medium potatoes (about 1 pound), scrubbed
            but not peeled
      6–8 cloves garlic, unpeeled
        1 cup "cream" substitute (see p. 40)
        ½ teaspoon ground coriander
        ¼ teaspoon freshly ground nutmeg
        ¼ teaspoon white pepper
        1 small onion, finely chopped
        2 egg whites, or 1 whole egg

Preheat oven to 350 degrees. Place potatoes and garlic in a
medium saucepan; add water to cover and cook until potatoes
are tender—about 30 minutes. Remove potatoes and garlic
from liquid with a slotted spoon, saving the broth. Peel the
potatoes or not, as you prefer. Mash potatoes with a fork;
remove peel from garlic, mash and add to potatoes. Mix together "cream," coriander, nutmeg and pepper; combine with
potato-garlic mixture.

Cook onion in ¼ cup broth saved from cooking potatoes.
When onion is tender, place onion, onion broth and egg
whites or whole egg in a blender or food processor; process
until onion is pureed. Mix onion with potato-garlic mixture.
Place this mixture in a lightly greased or nonstick 1½-quart
casserole. Bake for 30 minutes, or refrigerate at this point. If
the potatoes are prepared ahead and refrigerated, allow an
extra 5 minutes of baking time.

Makes 4 servings.

Potatoes and Vegetables with Seasoned Tofu Mayonnaise

1   cup Tofu Mayonnaise (see p. 36)
1   teaspoon minced fresh tarragon or ¼ teaspoon dried
⅛   teaspoon garlic powder
    dash freshly ground pepper
8   small red potatoes, cooked and chilled
1   small cauliflower, trimmed and separated into florets
8   green onions, trimmed
8   celery ribs, cut into 2-inch lengths
16 cherry tomatoes
16 whole mushrooms

Combine Tofu Mayonnaise, tarragon, garlic powder and pepper. Allow to stand for 15 to 20 minutes so flavors will blend. Meanwhile arrange the vegetables attractively on a platter. Place mayonnaise in a small bowl. Guests help themselves by dipping potatoes and vegetables in mayonnaise. An alternate serving suggestion is to cut vegetables into bite-size pieces and toss them lightly with mayonnaise mixture; serve on a platter lined with red leaf lettuce.

Makes 4 servings.

Tsimmes

Tsimmes has come to mean the overcomplication of a relatively simple situation—"she made a big *tsimmes* over changing her diet." Originally the word referred to a vegetable stew containing carrots that cooked until all the ingredients blended.

> 3 large sweet potatoes, scrubbed, sliced, then slices quartered
> 1 cup pitted whole prunes
> 2 whole oranges, thinly sliced
> 4 large carrots, sliced
> ½ teaspoon ground cardamom
> ½ teaspoon cinnamon
> 2 cups white grape juice, no sugar added

Preheat oven to 325 degrees. Combine sweet potatoes, prunes, oranges and carrots in a large covered casserole. Add spices to grape juice and pour over fruits and vegetables. Bake for 2 hours. Check occasionally to see if Tsimmes is too dry; if necessary, add more grape juice.

Makes 4 to 6 servings.

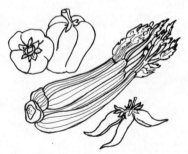

"Candied" Sweet Potatoes

   ½ cup dried apricots
   ½ cup dark raisins
   1 cup unsweetened apple juice
   4 medium sweet potatoes, scrubbed and trimmed
   1 tablespoon tapioca
1–2 tablespoons brandy (optional)
   1 cup unsweetened applesauce

Preheat oven to 350 degrees. Wash apricots and soak with raisins in apple juice for 1 hour. Steam sweet potatoes until tender. In a small saucepan combine tapioca with apricots, raisins and juice. Let mixture stand for 5 minutes; then bring to a boil over medium heat, stirring often. Remove from heat. Add brandy if desired and cool for 20 minutes.

Cut cooked sweet potatoes into ½-inch slices; mix with applesauce. Place this mixture in a 1½-quart casserole. Pour the apricot-raisin sauce over the top. Bake, uncovered, for 30 minutes.

Makes 6 servings.

Island Sweet Potatoes

> 4 large sweet potatoes
> One 20-ounce can crushed pineapple, no sugar added
> ¼ teaspoon ground ginger
> ¼ teaspoon grated nutmeg
> ½ teaspoon ground cinnamon
> 1 tablespoon dark rum (optional)

Preheat oven to 400 degrees. Scrub the sweet potatoes and prick them with a fork. Bake them for 1 hour or until tender when squeezed. Cut each potato in half and carefully remove pulp, leaving a ½-inch shell. Drain the pineapple and save the juice. Mash the sweet potato pulp with the pineapple, ½ cup of the juice, spices and rum if used. Pile mixture into reserved shells and return to oven. Reduce heat to 350 degrees and bake until heated through—about 15 minutes.

Makes 8 servings.

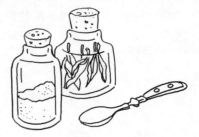

RICE

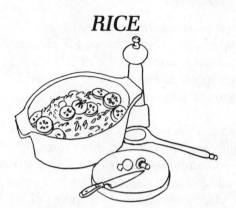

Experiment with different kinds of rice. Long-grain rice is dry and fluffy. Short-grain rice tends to be sticky. Brown rice, long or short, is chewy and nutty but takes longer to cook than white. Converted rice is a long-grain white that still retains many of the nutrients of the brown rice. Basmati rice is a newcomer to the market; either white or brown, it is flavorful and fluffy but more expensive than ordinary rice.

Rémoulade Rice

This cold salad goes well with seafood, picnic foods or any summer fare.

> 2 cups hot cooked converted rice (cook in water seasoned with 1 tablespoon cider vinegar, ¼ teaspoon paprika and ¼ teaspoon minced parsley)
> ½ cup drained whipped tofu, or ½ cup plain nonfat or low-fat yogurt
> 2 tablespoons catsup, no salt added
> ¼ teaspoon onion powder
> ¼ teaspoon dry mustard

  ¼ teaspoon paprika
  1 tablespoon finely chopped fresh parsley
  ¼ teaspoon tarragon
  ¼ teaspoon cayenne
     ground pepper to taste

Spoon rice into a deep bowl. Combine tofu, catsup and seasonings. Pour over hot rice and mix thoroughly. Chill.

To serve, mound seasoned rice on a platter and garnish with cold cooked or raw vegetables such as asparagus spears, sliced beets, cherry tomatoes or cucumber slices.

Makes 4 servings.

Peas and Mushroom Risotto

  1–2 cloves garlic, minced
   ½ pound fresh mushrooms, sliced
   1 tablespoon defatted, unsalted stock (see pp.
       25–28)
   1 cup Basmati or long-grain rice
   1 cup water
   1 cup white wine
      pinch of turmeric
   1 cup frozen peas, thawed but not cooked

Cook garlic and mushrooms in stock for 3 to 4 minutes or until soft but not browned. Raise heat and simmer to evaporate all but 1 teaspoon of liquid. Stir in rice and cook for several minutes. Blend in water, wine and turmeric; bring to a simmer. Stir once, then cover and let cook for 12 to 15 minutes. Taste to see that rice is tender. Stir in peas; cover and let stand for 1 to 2 minutes or until peas are warm.

This dish may be prepared ahead and refrigerated. Set rice-cooking pan in a larger pan of simmering water to reheat.

Makes 4 servings.

Fruited Rice

1–2 tablespoons defatted, unsalted stock (see pp. 25–28)
  1 small onion, chopped
  ⅓ cup raisins
  ⅓ cup chopped dried apricots
  ⅓ cup chopped water chestnuts (optional)
  1 cup Basmati or long-grain rice
  1 cup water
  1 cup white wine (sauterne is nice here)
  ½ teaspoon cinnamon
  ½ teaspoon coriander
    dash of white pepper

Heat stock in a large nonstick frying pan. Add onion and cook until lightly browned. Add fruit and water chestnuts. Stir in rice and cook on high heat for several minutes to coat grains of rice with liquid from onions and fruit. Combine water, wine and seasonings; pour over rice. Bring to a boil, stirring once. Lower the heat, cover and simmer for 12 to 15 minutes or until rice is tender and all stock has been absorbed.

Makes 4 servings.

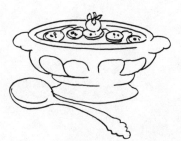

Dentist-Approved Desserts

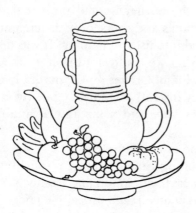

Our favorite dessert and the one we serve most frequently requires no recipe. It is simply fresh fruit in season. Sometimes we offer a bowl of whole fruits; at other times we prepare layers of colorful bites in a glass bowl. But when we have company or on special occasions when we want to show off, we turn to recipes designed to impress—not to flaunt the richness of our dessert but to show that elegant dishes like Bananas Flambé or Pears Fresco can still be low in fat, salt and sugar.

Bananas Flambé

We first tasted this dessert in an elegant restaurant in New Orleans. Using a chafing dish at the side of our table, the waiter melted a huge chunk of butter, to which he added a generous helping of brown sugar. When that was mixed together, he added two bananas, quartered. He turned the bananas around and around in the rich sauce until they were thoroughly coated and cooked through. Then he poured on orange liqueur and rum, and tipped the dish sideways so that the flame from the burner ignited the bananas. Quickly he spooned the bananas and sauce over the creamiest vanilla ice cream and served it to us, still flaming. It was delicious, but so sweet and rich that we could not finish it.

Our Bananas Flambé relies on the naturally occurring sugars in fruit juices instead of added sugar. By cooking in fruit juice concentrate, we avoid using any fat at all.

> ½ teaspoon cornstarch
> ½ cup orange juice, fresh or reconstituted
>   dash each cinnamon and freshly ground nutmeg
> 2 tablespoons frozen pineapple juice concentrate, no sugar added
> 2 bananas, cut into four long quarters
> ¼ cup rum

Combine cornstarch, orange juice and spices, and set aside. Place the pineapple juice concentrate and the quartered bananas in a shallow pan with a long handle. Cook at the table over an alcohol flame or over medium heat on the range until bananas are soft and heated through, turning them to coat all sides. Pour the orange juice mixture over the bananas and simmer until sauce thickens. Hold the rum in a ladle above the bananas for just a moment to heat it, then pour it over the bananas. Flame the rum by tipping it toward the burner (as described) at the table, or with a match at the range. Serve immediately. This dessert is so good it can be eaten just as it is, but if you wish to put something under it to contrast with its richness, use vanilla ice milk or a slice of unfrosted angel food cake.

Makes 4 servings.

Pears Fresco

The cream in the original of this recipe was a rich egg-milk custard combined with 1 cup whipping cream and sweetened with ½ cup sugar. By eliminating egg yolks (3), whole milk and whipping cream, we greatly decrease the cholesterol and fat. This dessert would be especially good for those on a low-salt diet, since our "cream," particularly if it is made with dry cottage cheese, is very low in sodium.

4–6 firm, ripe pears such as Bosc
3 tablespoons orange-flavored liqueur
1½ cups "cream" (see p. 40)
3 tablespoons pineapple or orange juice concentrate
2 egg whites
1 teaspoon vanilla
1 tablespoon finely chopped almonds

Peel the pears, cut them in even slices and sprinkle with the liqueur. Cover. Mix together "cream" and fruit juice concentrate. Cover and allow to stand for several hours so that flavors blend. About 2 hours before serving beat egg whites until soft peaks form; stir in vanilla. Fold egg whites into "cream." Layer the "cream" and pears in a deep bowl. Cover and chill. Sprinkle with nuts just before serving.

Makes 4 to 6 servings.

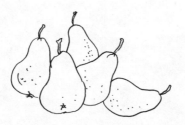

No-Bake Pineapple "Cream" Dessert

This one is for cheesecake lovers! We like it best made with our ricotta cream substitute, but you can use any one of our "creams" successfully.

One 20-ounce can crushed pineapple
2 tablespoons (2 packages) unflavored gelatin
2 cups "cream" (see p. 40)
1½ teaspoons vanilla
1 teaspoon orange extract
1 teaspoon grated orange rind
2 egg whites
sliced strawberries or kiwi fruit, as garnish

Drain pineapple; save juice. Measure 1½ cups pineapple juice into a small saucepan. Sprinkle with gelatin and let soften for one minute. Bring to a simmer and heat until gelatin dissolves. Cool. In a blender or food processor, combine "cream," vanilla, orange extract, rind and pineapple; blend for 1 minute. Pour mixture into a large bowl. Stir in gelatin and refrigerate until mixture begins to thicken.

Beat egg whites until stiff. Fold into pineapple mixture. Pour into 9- or 10-inch pie pan or spring form. Chill until firm. Decorate the top with strawberries that have been marinated in pineapple concentrate or fruit-flavored liqueur, or top with sliced ripe kiwi fruit.

Makes 8 servings.

Sparkling Strawberries

> 2 cups unsweetened white grape juice
> 1 envelope (1 tablespoon) unflavored gelatin
> One 16-ounce package frozen strawberries, no sugar
>   added, or 2 cups fresh whole or halved
>   strawberries
> sweetened "cream" (optional—recipe follows)

Place grape juice in a medium saucepan. Sprinkle gelatin on juice and let soften for 3 to 4 minutes. Cook over medium heat, stirring constantly, until gelatin is dissolved. Remove from heat. Pour into a glass bowl and chill until mixture begins to thicken. Fold in berries. Chill until set. Top with sweetened "cream," if desired.

Makes 4 to 5 servings.

SWEETENED "CREAM"

> ½ cup "cream" substitute (see p. 40)
> 2 teaspoons frozen juice concentrate

Beat cream for 2 to 3 minutes and stir in juice concentrate.

Parisian Berries

> 4 cups whole fresh berries
> 2 tablespoons orange-flavored liqueur
> 1 cup nonfat milk
> 1 tablespoon cornstarch or arrowroot
> 2 tablespoons pineapple juice concentrate
> 1½ teaspoons vanilla
> 2 egg whites
> ⅛ teaspoon cream of tartar

Marinate berries in liqueur and set aside. Pour milk into a small saucepan; stir in cornstarch and add juice concentrate. Cook on low heat until mixture boils, then simmer until thickened, stirring constantly. Pour into a bowl. Let cool, then add vanilla.

Combine egg whites and cream of tartar; beat until stiff. Fold egg whites into sauce. Stir in berries. Serve in a clear glass bowl or individual wineglasses.

Makes 8 servings.

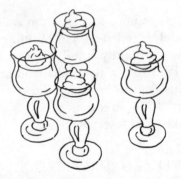

Pumpkin Parfait

What would Thanksgiving be without as pumpkin dessert! You can serve this parfait as described here, or layer the pumpkin and ricotta mixtures to make a striped dessert.

    1   egg yolk
    ½   cup frozen apple juice concentrate
    1¼ cups pumpkin, canned or cooked
    ½   teaspoon ground ginger
    ½   teaspoon ground cinnamon
    ½   teaspoon freshly grated nutmeg
    ¼   teaspoon ground cloves
    1   envelope (1 tablespoon) unflavored gelatin
    ¼   cup cold water
    2   egg whites

Beat the egg yolk with the apple juice concentrate. Add pumpkin and spices. Cook in a double boiler until thick.

Soften gelatin in cold water; stir into pumpkin mixture. Chill until partially set. Beat egg whites until stiff. Fold into pumpkin mixture until no trace of white shows. Spoon pumpkin into tall parfait glasses and chill. Serve with Ricotta Topping (recipe follows).

Makes 4 servings.

RICOTTA TOPPING

    1 cup skim milk ricotta cheese
    2 tablespoons frozen apple juice concentrate

Whip both ingredients together until smooth and creamy.

Makes 1 cup.

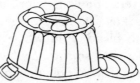

Gelatin Mold Filled with Fruit

      1 package (1 tablespoon) unflavored gelatin
      2 tablespoons water
      1 tablespoon lemon juice
    ⅛ teaspoon oil
  One 15½-ounce can crushed pineapple, drained
      1 cup nonfat yogurt
      2 ripe bananas, pureed

In a small bowl combine gelatin, water and lemon juice. Stir; set this bowl in a container of boiling water. Grease a 3- to 4-cup ring mold with ⅛ teaspoon oil. In a large bowl combine pineapple and yogurt. Stir well. Mix in the banana. Add gelatin mixture. Stir. Pour into mold and refrigerate until firm. Remove from mold and fill the center with fresh fruit.

Makes 4 servings.

Whole Wheat Apple Kuchen

     2 packages dry yeast
     1 cup warm water
     ½ cup apple juice concentrate, thawed
     ½ cup nonfat dry milk
     2 tablespoons unsalted corn oil margarine
     2 egg whites, lightly beaten
     2 cups whole wheat flour
2–2½ cups unbleached white flour

Combine yeast with warm water in the large bowl of an electric mixer. Stir with a fork until dissolved. Add apple juice concentrate, dry milk, margarine and egg whites. Beat at low speed to blend. Add whole wheat flour, ½ cup at a time, blending until smooth. By hand, stir in enough white flour to make a soft, workable dough. Knead on a floured surface for 10 minutes, until dough is smooth and elastic. Place dough in a warm, greased bowl, turning to coat the top. Cover with a towel and let rise in a warm place until double in size—about 1½ hours.

Meanwhile, prepare filling (recipe follows) and set aside.

Preheat oven to 350 degrees. When dough has doubled, punch down, cover and let rest for 10 minutes more. Divide the dough into two equal parts. Roll one part into a 13-by-9-inch rectangle. Spread half the filling over the dough. Roll up, starting with the long side. Place seam side down on a nonstick baking sheet. Shape the kuchen by making cuts into each side of the roll at 1-inch intervals, leaving about 1 inch uncut down the middle. (To avoid damaging the nonstick surface, use a plastic knife or scissors.) Lift the cut sections, being careful not to tear each from the middle. Twist each section enough to expose the spiral pattern and lay each section on top of the one behind, like fallen dominoes. Repeat assembly with the second half of the dough and the remaining filling. Cover both kuchen and let dough rise until double—30 to 45 minutes. Bake for 25 to 30 minutes.

FILLING

    1 teaspoon cornstarch
    ½ cup unsweetened apple juice, not concentrated
    2 cups chopped apples
    1 teaspoon cinnamon
    1 tablespoon lemon juice
    ½ cup raisins
    1 teaspoon vanilla

Stir cornstarch into apple juice and set aside. Combine apples, cinnamon, lemon juice and raisins in a small saucepan. Bring to a boil and simmer for 5 minutes. Add apple juice to apples and cook over medium heat, stirring constantly, until mixture boils. Boil for 1 minute. Remove from heat; add vanilla.

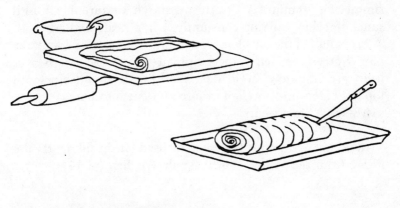

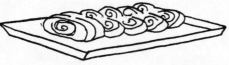

Oatbar Crumbles

    2 cups rolled oats
    ½ cup whole wheat pastry flour
    ½ cup nonfat dry milk
    1 teaspoon cinnamon
    ¼ cup frozen apple juice concentrate, thawed
    ¼ cup safflower oil
  One 1-pound can pears, no sugar added
    1 tablespoon cornstarch

Preheat oven to 375 degrees. Blend oatmeal in a blender or
food processor until it resembles flour. In a medium mixing
bowl, combine oats, flour, dry milk and cinnamon. Mix together juice concentrate and oil; stir into oat-flour mixture
until dough holds together. Set dough aside and prepare filling.

Drain pears, reserving juice. Mix 2 tablespoons juice with
the cornstarch. Heat remaining juice in a small saucepan;
simmer for 10 minutes. Stir in cornstarch mixture. Heat until
sauce thickens, stirring constantly. Chop pears and add.

Press half of the oat-flour dough into a nonstick 8-inch cake
pan. Spread on pear sauce. Spread remaining dough over
fruit, pressing down well. Bake for 30 to 35 minutes or until
top is golden brown. Cool in pan and cut into bars.

Makes 12 to 15 bars.

VARIATION: Any fruit sauce can be used for the filling; try the
filling from the Whole Wheat Apple Kuchen (p. 144).

Pear Cookies

There are two kinds of dried fruits. One is dried naturally in the sun and tends to be very hard. The other has been treated with a preservative, which produces a softer fruit. When we made these cookies, we used naturally dried pears that were stiff and hard and required a long soaking time—about two hours! You might want to start such pears soaking the night before you make these cookies.

>   1 cup coarsely chopped dried pears
> 1/3 cup frozen juice concentrate
>   1 tablespoon fruit-flavored liqueur (we used
>   Kirschberry)
>   1 tablespoon cocoa
> 1/3 cup uncooked oatmeal

Soak chopped pears in juice concentrate and liqueur until soft enough to puree in a food processor or blender. Puree fruit mixture and combine with cocoa and oatmeal. The mixture will be sticky, but it should be firm enough to be rolled into a ball. Add more oatmeal as necessary, a tablespoon at a time. Roll by teaspoonfuls in your hands to make balls about 3/4 inch in diameter. These cookies taste even better after they stand overnight.

Makes 18 cookies.

Baked Apples Stuffed with Dried Fruits

                6   large baking apples
                3   dried figs, chopped
                3   dried dates, chopped
                2   tablespoons chopped raisins
              ½   teaspoon freshly grated ginger
                1   cup unsweetened apple juice

Preheat oven to 350 degrees. Wash apples. Scoop out the cores. Combine dried fruits and ginger. Stuff apples with mix. Set apples in a pan so that they fit snugly. Pour in juice. Bake for 45 minutes or until apples are soft, basting frequently. Serve warm.

Makes 6 servings.

Winter Mélange

This fruit combination is a lovely gift to bring to a hostess. Prepare it in a glass apothecary jar with a secure lid.

                1   cup dried dates, pitted and cut in half
                1   cup dried apricot halves
                1   lemon with peel, cut in thin slices
                1   cup white raisins
              ½   teaspoon ground cardamom
                1   cup boiling water
                1   tablespoon brandy (optional)

Combine all the fruits and the cardamom in an attractive glass bowl or jar. Pour boiling water over all. Cover and let stand at room temperature until cool, stirring occasionally. Refrigerate. If desired, stir in brandy just before serving or giving as a gift.

Makes 6 servings.

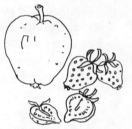

Quick Sherbet

In the summertime when there is often a surplus of fresh fruit, a quick sherbet is a welcome relief from the heat and the monotony.

    2–3 cups fresh fruit
    2–3 tablespoons frozen fruit juice concentrate
           (amount depends on sweetness of fruit)

Wash fruit. Cut into 1- to 2-inch chunks. Place on a plate and set in freezer until hard. Just before serving, puree the frozen fruit in a food processor; add fruit juice concentrate to taste and process until mixture is of sherbet consistency.

Makes 4 servings.

Frozen Fruit Fantasy

If you love to experiment with new combinations of flavors, this dessert needn't ever taste the same twice. You mix fruit puree with fruit juice concentrate and seasonings. You can choose your fruit, vary the juice concentrate and play with seasonings. For example, we tried banana puree with pineapple juice concentrate and orange rind.

It takes almost two cups of cut fruit to make one cup of puree. Bananas can be mashed with a fork; other fruits do better in a blender or a food processor. Some berries and grapes will need to be strained.

```
1  tablespoon (1 envelope) unflavored gelatin
2  tablespoons cold water
1  tablespoon lemon juice
1  cup fresh fruit puree
1  teaspoon grated lemon or orange rind, or
     ½ teaspoon ground ginger, cinnamon
     or cardamom
2  tablespoons frozen fruit juice concentrate or
     honey
2  cups plain low-fat or nonfat yogurt
2  egg whites
```

Soften gelatin in cold water for 2 or 3 minutes. Combine gelatin, lemon juice, fruit puree, grated rind or seasoning, fruit juice concentrate and yogurt and mix thoroughly. Freeze until crystals begin to form around the edges. Beat egg whites until stiff. Break up the yogurt mix with a spoon and then beat with an electric mixer until smooth. Fold in beaten egg whites. Freeze until firm. About 30 minutes before serving, remove from freezer to refrigerator to allow dessert to soften.

Makes 2 to 2½ cups.

APPENDIXES

Appendix A

Fat, Cholesterol and Sodium Content of Common Foods

FOOD	AMOUNT	TOTAL FAT (grams)	CHOLESTEROL (milligrams)	SODIUM (milligrams)
whole milk (3.5% fat)	1 cup	8.5	34	122
2%-fat milk	1 cup	4.9	19	145
1%-fat milk	1 cup	2.6	10	123
nonfat milk (skim)	1 cup	.6	5	130
evaporated skim milk	½ cup	.3	5	147
nonfat instant dry milk	1⅓ cups or 3.2-ounce envelope to make one quart	.7	17	499
creamed (4% fat) cottage cheese	1 cup unpacked	9.5	31	850
low-fat (2% fat) cottage cheese	1 cup unpacked	4.4	19	918
dry-curd cottage cheese	1 cup unpacked	.6	10	19
ricotta cheese	½ cup	16.1	63	104
ricotta cheese, part skim milk	½ cup	9.8	38	155
plain yogurt	1 cup	7.4	29	105
plain low-fat yogurt	1 cup	3.5	14	159
plain nonfat yogurt	1 cup	.4	4	174
tofu	1 cup	10	0	16

Food	Amount			
heavy cream, unwhipped	1 cup	88.1	326	89
half and half	1 cup	27.8	89	98
sour cream	1 cup	48	102	123
cream cheese	3-ounce package	29.6	93	251
cheddar cheese	1 ounce shredded	9.4	30	176
mozzarella, low-moisture, part skim	1 ounce	4.8	15	150
sapsago	1 ounce	2.6	unavailable	363–510
butter, salted	1 tablespoon	11.3	35	138
butter, unsalted	1 tablespoon	11.3	35	1
margarine, salted	1 tablespoon	11.3	0	138
margarine, unsalted	1 tablespoon	11.3	0	1
safflower oil	1 tablespoon	14	0	0
olive oil	1 tablespoon	14	0	0
chicken egg, whole	1 egg	5.6	274	69
chicken egg, yolk	1 yolk	5.6	272	8
chicken egg, white	1 white	trace	0	50
chicken, meat and skin (cooked)	½ breast	7.6	83	69
chicken, meat only (cooked)	½ breast	3.07	73	63
ground beef, lean	3 to 3½ ounces	11.3	70	50
ground beef, regular	3 to 3½ ounces	20.3	70	50

NOTE: These figures are based on *Composition of Foods*, Agriculture Handbook Nos. 8, 8-1 and 8-5, U.S. Department of Agriculture, Washington, D.C.

Appendix B

Calories and Nutrients of Selected Foods

FOOD	AMOUNT	CALORIES	CALCIUM (mg)	VITAMIN A (IU)	IRON (mg)	VITAMIN C (mg)	POTASSIUM (mg)
heavy cream substitute	1 cup	821	154	3499	.07	1.38	179
"creams": skim milk							
ricotta	1 cup	371	433	1067	1.13	trace	433
2% cottage cheese	1 cup	234	268	162	.41	trace	362
dry curd cheese	1 cup	154	159	48	.38	trace	192
tofu topping	1 cup	252	245.5	350	4.31	42	600
banana	1 medium	101	10	230	.8	12	440
banana, mashed	1 cup	191	18	430	1.6	23	833
apple	1 medium	96	12	150	.5	7	172
orange	1 medium	87	9	170	.2	52	164

pear, Bosc	1 medium	86	11	30	.4	6	183
raisins	1 cup	419	90	30	5.1	1	1106
dates, chopped	1 cup	488	105	90	5.3	0	1153
pineapple, crushed, canned in its own juice	1 cup	130	36	145	.9	23	333
carrots, raw, shredded	½ cup	15	23	3965	.25	3	123
honey	1 tablespoon	64	1	0	.1	0	11
sugar	1 tablespoon	46	0	0	0	0	trace
frozen apple juice concentrate	1 tablespoon	29	3.7	0	.16	trace	77
frozen orange juice concentrate	1 tablespoon	28	5.5	135	.06	30	119
blackstrap molasses	1 tablespoon	43	137	0	3.2	0	585

Index

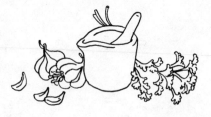

Join the millions of Americans who are turning to nutrition as the way to better health, with Perigee guides by the foremost experts in the field!

THE BARBARA KRAUS 30-DAY CHOLESTEROL PROGRAM
A Diet and Exercise Plan for Lowering Your Cholesterol
by Barbara Kraus

Don't just count your cholesterol intake—do something about it! Whether you're young or old, or have a serious problem or want to prevent having one, here are practical suggestions for a low-fat, high-fiber diet that will help you reduce your serum cholesterol.

THE DICTIONARY OF SODIUM, FATS, AND CHOLESTEROL
Second Edition
by Barbara Kraus

No matter what diet you're on, you can instantly calculate the sodium, fat, and cholesterol content of everything you eat, with the completely revised edition of this ground-breaking book. Alphabetical listings of 10,000 brand names and basic foods are cross-referenced for easy use.

THE BARBARA KRAUS CHOLESTEROL COUNTER
by Barbara Kraus

Here is a concise guide to the cholesterol content of nearly 2,000 foods—from eggs and meats, grains and fruits, to take-out foods and brand-name packaged foods.

THE BARBARA KRAUS CALORIE COUNTER
by Barbara Kraus

This completely updated edition of the definitive calorie counter for dieters and health advocates provides counts for basic foods from abalone to zwieback as well as the latest formulations of brand-name packaged foods and beverages.

THE PEOPLE'S NUTRITION ENCYCLOPEDIA
by Lynne S. Hill, M.S., R.D.

Based on recently released data from the USDA, this comprehensive one-volume guide breaks down the ten most frequently asked-about food values—calories, calcium, cholesterol, fat, sodium, fiber, iron, carbohydrates, protein, and potassium—of over 9,000 basic and brand-name foods.

THE COLUMBIA ENCYCLOPEDIA OF NUTRITION
from the Institute of Human Nutrition, Columbia University College of Physicians and Surgeons
Compiled and edited by Myron Winick, M.D.

From general entries on adolescence, pregnancy, and cancer to the specifics on amino acids, caffeine, and vitamins, this up-to-date master reference covers every aspect of nutrition as it relates to diet, disease, stress, sports, mental health, and more.

NEW LOW BLOOD SUGAR AND YOU
by Carlton Fredericks, Ph.D.

Do you suffer from anxiety, irritability, exhaustion, headaches, indecisiveness, insomnia, or forgetfulness? If the answer is yes, you, like millions of other Americans, may suffer from hypoglycemia (low blood sugar). Now the nation's number-one authority on this hidden disease tells how you can control it by changing your diet.

HOLD THE FAT, SUGAR & SALT
by Goldie Silverman and Jacqueline Williams

Here's the first—and only—cookbook that includes easy-to-follow cooking techniques plus over 100 mouth-watering recipes for transforming all your favorite dishes into nutritional treats that will pamper your palate without hindering your health.

Ordering is easy and convenient. Just call **1-800-631-8571** or send your order to:

The Putnam Publishing Group
390 Murray Hill Parkway, Dept. B
East Rutherford, NJ 07073

Also available at your local bookstore or wherever paperbacks are sold.

		PRICE	
		U.S.	CANADA
____ The Barbara Kraus 30-Day Cholesterol Program	399-51508	$ 6.95	$ 9.25
____ The Dictionary of Sodium, Fats, and Cholesterol	399-51572	12.95	16.95
____ The Barbara Kraus Cholesterol Counter	399-51134	6.95	9.25
____ The Barbara Kraus Calorie Counter	399-51222	6.95	9.25
____ The People's Nutrition Encyclopedia	399-51289	11.95	15.75
____ The Columbia Encyclopedia of Nutrition	399-51573	12.95	16.95
____ New Low Blood Sugar and You	399-51087	7.95	10.50
____ Hold the Fat, Sugar & Salt	399-51073	7.95	10.50

Subtotal $_____

*Postage & handling $_____

Sales Tax $_____
(CA, NJ, NY, PA)

*Postage & handling:
$2.00 for 1 book, 50¢
for each additional book
up to a maximum of $4.50

Total Amount Due $_____
Payable in U.S. Funds
(No cash orders accepted)

_____

Please send me the titles I've checked above.
Enclosed is my ☐ check   ☐ money order
Please charge my ☐ Visa   ☐ MasterCard   ☐ American Express
(Minimum order for charge cards is $10.00.)
Card # _____Expiration date _____

Signature as on charge card _____

Name _____

Address _____

City_____State _____ Zip _____

Please allow six weeks for delivery. Prices subject to change without notice.